INDOOR ROWING
for Fitness and Competition

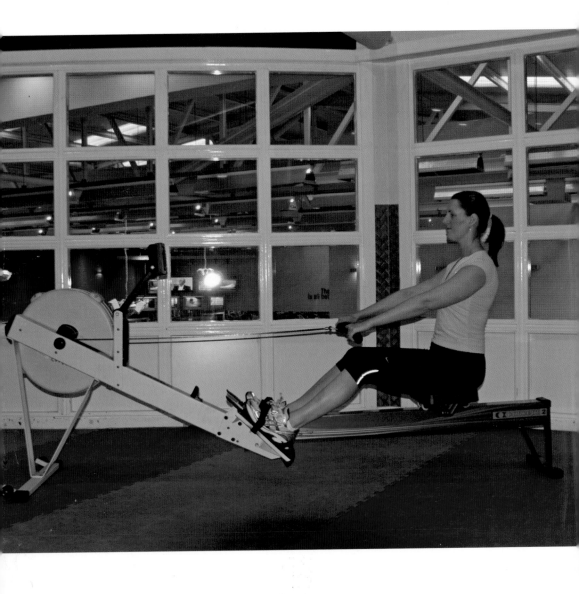

INDOOR ROWING
for Fitness and Competition

Darryl Wilkinson

THE CROWOOD PRESS

First published in 2010 by
The Crowood Press Ltd
Ramsbury, Marlborough
Wiltshire SN8 2HR

www.crowood.com

British Library Cataloguing-in-Publication Data
A catalogue record for this book is available from the British Library.

ISBN 978 1 84797 191 3

Disclaimer
Please note that the author and the publisher of this book are not responsible
in any manner whatsoever for any damage or injury or adverse outcome of
any kind that may result from practising, or applying, the principles, ideas,
techniques and/or following the instructions/information described in this
publication. Since the physical activities covered in this book may be too
strenuous in nature for some readers to engage in safely, it is essential that
a doctor be consulted before undertaking any training, exercises or indoor
rowing. The chapter entitled 'Injury and Injury Prevention' is intended as
a basic helpful guide to common indoor rowing injuries and it is not intended
to replace professional medical diagnosis or treatment. Its aim is to help
reduce the risk of injury and the exercises described should not be
undertaken by individuals suffering with an injury.

Although this book contains references to particular types and models of
rowing machine, this does not signify that those products are endorsed by the
publishers.

Designed and typeset by Focus Publishing,
Sevenoaks, Kent

Printed and bound in Malaysia by Times Offset (M) Sdn Bhd

Contents

Acknowledgements

I would like to thank everyone who has been part of this project and helped to turn my vision into reality. Specifically, I would like to mention the following: The Crowood Press, who have turned this book into what it is; to all the knowledgeable and understanding staff at Concept2 UK and US for their help and advice, especially Suzanne Hudson who has answered all of my questions; and finally to all the professional staff at Fitness First and their excellent facilities, especially Derek Crawford, who has been an inspiration through my fitness career. I am grateful to so many others who have helped me be who I am, but I am especially grateful to my wife, Sharon Wilkinson, who has always believed in me and makes me want to be myself and better.

1 The Journey from Outdoor to Indoor

Rowing as Sport

The earliest known records of oars and rowing date back to Egypt in the fourth millennium BC. From then on, rowing played an important role in trade and commerce for thousands of years. The idea of rowing for exercise or as a competitive sport, however, was not common before 1800, and it was not until the late twentieth century that indoor rowing, using static, land-based machines, emerged as a sport in its own right.

One of the oldest surviving boat races is the Doggett's Coat and Badge, named after the prize – a scarlet coat and a silver badge. The race was founded in 1715 by Thomas Doggett, who organized the event himself every year on the River Thames up to his death in 1721. The four-and-a-half mile (7.25km) race started from London Bridge and finished at the Swan Inn at Chelsea. Except that the Swan Inn has long gone, the race route has remained the same ever since. Until the early 1870s the race was always against the tide (usually taking the unfortunate rower around two hours to complete), but now the race is rowed with the tide, making it more manageable for all competitors. It takes place at the end of July every year and can be viewed from anywhere along the route.

Probably the most famous boat race is the University Boat Race, which runs on the Thames every spring. The original idea for a race between crews from Oxford and Cambridge universities started with two friends who had met at Harrow School. Charles Wordsworth, a nephew of the poet William Wordsworth, was a student at Oxford, while Charles Merivale was at Cambridge. The first challenge was sent by Cambridge to Oxford in March 1829; by tradition, the loser of the previous year now challenges the opposition to a re-match. The first race took place at Henley-on-Thames and was such a success that the townspeople decided to organize their own regatta. It was some years before the universities could agree on a new course. In 1836 they raced from Westminster to Putney, but, due to overcrowding, the race was later moved six miles upstream to start from Putney. Since 1856 the race has become an annual event (only excluding the war years). The modern version of the Boat Race is a major international event, drawing in millions of television viewers from around the world and up to 250,000 spectators on the banks of the Thames from Putney to Mortlake.

From the early nineteenth century rowing became more than just a means to get from one place to another or transport goods. Boat races slowly became popular throughout America, Australia and England. It was not until the mid-nineteenth century that the sport spread to mainland Europe, with the foundation of the Ghent Rowing Club in Belgium in 1846 and the Gothenburg Rowing Club in Sweden in 1851. The first modern rowing races were introduced in England as competitions between professional watermen, who were an essential part of early London life and provided a 'taxi' service along the River Thames, using a small boat called a wherry or skiff. The awful state of the roads, both the narrow, jam-packed London streets and in the surrounding country, meant that the Thames was one of the most convenient ways to get about the city. The watermen competed for prizes provided by the wealthy owners of riverside houses. Between 1800 and 1900 races of this type became popular throughout Great Britain and it was not long before the sport spread to other rivers and people started to organize their own races. Rowing regattas were introduced and continued throughout the twentieth century, but it wasn't until the second half of the twentieth century that indoor rowing started to make its appearance as a competitive activity.

The first rowing machines of various types were patented from the mid-nineteenth century. The Narragansett, based on a hydraulic action and built by the Narragansett Machine Company in Providence, Rhode Island, was the first choice for many rowers from 1900 to about 1960, when an Australian company introduced the ergometer (from Greek: ergon, 'work'). This was designed to measure work capacity with leather straps applying a resistance to a flywheel. Early examples suffered from the drawback that atmospheric conditions could seriously reduce the reliability of the machine. By the 1970s, however, this problem had been solved by Gamut Engineering in northern California. The Gamut ergometer had arms that swivelled around a fixed axis and was very popular with competitive rowers until the early 1980s. It was then that indoor rowing took a huge step forward. The early forms of ergometer were usually very large, as well as very expensive and in constant need of maintenance. It was time for change. The Concept2 Indoor Rower, introduced in the early 1980s, has since become the pre-eminent indoor rowing machine and remains the main rower used for many of the indoor rowing competitions held today.

The Dreissigackers and the Concept2

The innovation that Peter and Dick Dreissigacker introduced in their Concept2 is its use of air as the braking system, so helping to simulate the water resistance that outdoor rowers experience. The Dreissigackers also developed a monitor that provided the user with feedback on every stroke. This was of crucial importance and set the Concept2 apart from its predecessors. It was these developments that resulted in the launch of indoor racing worldwide.

The Dreissigacker brothers were both keen rowers. Although they were not successful at the US national trials for the 1976 Olympic Games, the effort they had devoted to designing their own rowing oars was to pay off. Starting with carbon fibre oars, they founded a business to design and build rowing equipment. The company, based in Vermont, later expanded to develop many different types of rowing equipment for both outdoor and indoor use. Before the end of the decade, many colleges and universities were using the Dreissigacker oars for competitions.

The brothers had always dreamed of being able to continue rowing during the long winter months; one of their first inventions involved a bicycle nailed to the floor with a pull chain attached to it. In 1981 they developed the first Concept2 indoor rowing machine, which was mainly produced out of bicycle parts. It was widely known as the Model A. Each of the four models of the Concept2 that has followed has shown a dramatical improvement on its predecessor.

It was not long before the brothers moved into larger premises to meet the overwhelming demand for the Model A. The Model B rower, developed in 1986, was a much safer design than the Model A. It included a flywheel cover, had a more natural rowing movement, as well as a performance monitor that provided the user with the necessary workout details, updating the screen with every stroke.

The Model C rower followed in 1993. The new machine had a more streamlined appearance and it was not long before the Model C rower was being used in both health clubs and for home fitness. The Model D version of the Concept2, released in 2003, was quieter in operation performance and had a better range of damper levels and an impact-resistant flywheel cover. Its improved performance monitor removed all the paperwork that was once involved with monitoring workouts. This was achieved by developing what was known as a C2 log card, which allowed users to download their workouts to a computer. Workouts saved in this way could be started at the push of a button, instead of the user having to go through the hassle of entering the details every time. The Model E version, introduced in 2006, features a heavy-duty construction and an improved performance monitor. Improvements to the design mean that the parts are more accessible for cleaning, so reducing the risk of rust.

The Common Types of Rowing Machines

Despite the ubiquity of the Concept2, there is nonetheless plenty of choice when it comes to choosing an indoor rowing machine that suits your needs you. The available models may be divided into four categories:

Magnetic rowers. Magnetic-based rowing machines are renowned for their quietness during use. For resistance, the magnetic rower utilizes a magnetic brake system that produces no friction, greatly reducing the noise levels generated.

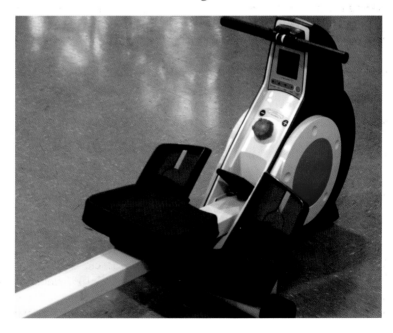

The magnetic rower is great for a quiet workout.

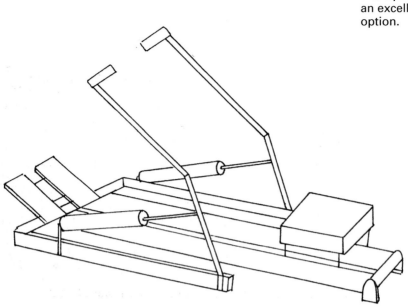

The hydraulic rower is an excellent low-cost option.

Hydraulic rowers. Hydraulic-based rowing machines are a smarter option if you feel space is a concern, or if you are on a tight budget. Hydraulic rowers produce their resistance from the amount of air or fluid that is compressed within a cylinder or piston; on most models this is adjustable. Hydraulic-based rowing machines are among the lowest cost options.

Water rowers. Water-based rowers are quickly becoming more popular. They mostly have a wooden frame, which can reduce the levels of mechanical vibration often found in other forms of indoor rowing machine. The water rower is designed to imitate the feeling of a boat moving through the water and the resistance is varied according to how much water is placed in the tank.

Flywheel rowers. Flywheel-based rowing machines, such as the Concept2, are also designed to closely simulate rowing in water. Resistance for the flywheel machine is provided by air passing through the machine as the user rows, spinning the flywheel that has fan blades attached. Using air as the resistance provides the user with a smooth continuous stroke.

The Future of Indoor Rowing

Outdoor rowing was one of the original sports included in the modern Olympic Games, and during the twentieth century it evolved into one of the most popular sports in the world. The introduction of technologically advanced indoor rowing machines added a new dimension to the sport. The popularity of both outdoor and indoor rowing continues to increase every year. The benefits of using an indoor rowing machine for sports training, fitness training and general health training has become more evident as our understanding of the science of fitness and health has advanced.

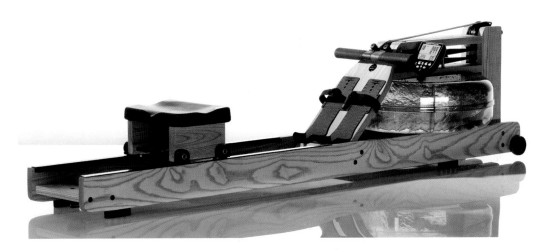

The water rower gives the user a realistic feel. (Courtesy of WaterRower UK Ltd)

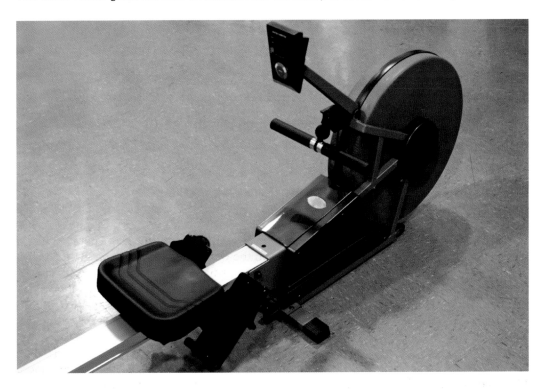

The flywheel rower is the most popular form of indoor rower.

2 Understanding the Competition Rower

Concept2 (C2) set the standard for affordable, durable and reliable indoor rowing machines. Even though other varieties of indoor ergometer have since been marketed, Concept2 is still the dominant brand in indoor rowing worldwide. The British, European and World Championships all use equipment of this type. Since it is by far the most popular machine in rowing clubs, fitness clubs and schools, both in the UK and elsewhere, the Concept2 indoor rowing machine will be referred to constantly throughout this book.

Concept2 Indoor Rower

When you first come to use a Concept2 indoor rowing machine you do not need to worry about having to operate any complicated computers before you start to exercise, since the performance monitor fitted to every model has an easy-to-follow workout display. Before you learn about each of the various performance monitors currently available, however, it is important to understand the basics of the Concept2 indoor rowing machine.

Unlike other cardiovascular machines you may have used in the gym, such as bikes, steppers and treadmills, Concept2 rowers do not have a preset resistance. Instead, the resistance on the rower is measured by how hard you can physically pull the bar and accelerate the rowing machine's flywheel during each rowing stoke. At the side of the fan cage there is a damper level, controlled by a lever that can be moved from a range of one to ten. This regulates what is known as the drag factor. When the lever is set to the lowest level (level one), less air passes through the fan of the rowing machine, resulting in a decreased rate of drag; as the lever is moved through the higher levels, up to level ten, more air passes through the fan, resulting in an increased rate of drag that makes the workout feel physically tougher. When you first use an indoor rowing machine it is a common mistake to believe you will get a more effective workout if you push the damper level up to the highest level. Do not be tempted to start too high, however, because this will only result in bad technique and you will not get the most out of your workout. Generally, the smaller and lighter you are, the more you would benefit from setting the damper level at a lower number (one to five). Heavier and stronger users would benefit from setting the damper level at a higher number (from six upwards).

Drag Factor

The performance monitor can be set to display a number known as the drag factor (displayed by default as 100 at level one and 220 at level ten). These figures can vary slightly, though, depending on the amount of dirt and dust that might have collected within the fan cage. If you want to simulate the feel of outdoor rowing, start by setting the damper level at the side to give a drag factor of between 130 and 140. There is always an element of trial and error in finding a drag factor that is comfortable for you and that you

The Concept2 rower is the choice for all major competitions.

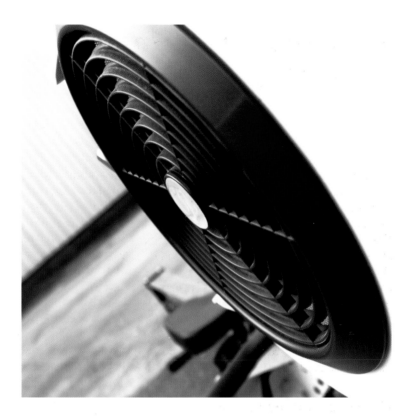

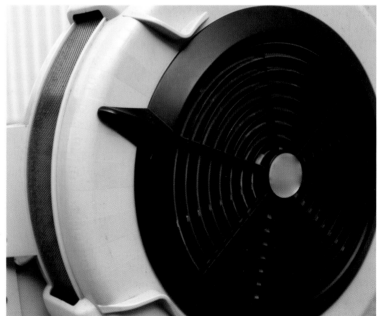

The 1–10 damper level scale will help you find the drag factor.

can maintain with a smooth and effective rowing stroke, but if you are in doubt this is a good level at which to start. It is also a good tip to remember what drag factor is best suited to you, since different indoor rowing machines can vary depending on their age and how regularly they are cleaned.

Performance Monitors

Performance monitors on Concept2 machines are designed to be self-explanatory, but there are some important differences between the different models you many encounter.

Performance Monitor 2 (PM2)

The PM2 is one of concept2's earlier designs, but is still a popular choice for many small gyms and homes. The performance monitor automatically starts up when you begin to row. The display provides information on five different aspects of the workout.

- Elapsed Time. The total time of your workout on the rowing machine.
- Stroke Rate. Shown in strokes per minute (spm), which is constantly updated with every stroke.
- Output. Shows how hard the individual has pulled on the last stroke. The output may be displayed as pace/500m, calories/hour or as watts.
- Total Output. Displays the total output since the start of the session as either average pace, metres, calories or watts.
- Heart rate. Shows the individual's heart rate in beats per minute (bpm). This section will only work if a heart rate interface is attached to the rowing machine and the user is wearing a chest-belt transmitter.

The PM2 also has four preset workouts: preset time duration, preset distance, timed intervals and distance intervals. After the session the user can review the workout performance by pushing the recall button. Additional options are available when two buttons are held down at the same time.

- Customize Splits for Time. To set time splits, press the ready and time buttons together, use the set digits buttons to set the split time and then press the ready button when finished.
- Customize Splits for Distance. To set distance splits, press the ready and metres buttons together, use the set digits buttons to set the split distance and then press the ready button when finished.
- Turn Splits On/Off. To display the split performance of the workout, press the ready and recall buttons together. The split score will be displayed for five seconds before returning back to the normal display.
- Display Drag Factor. To display the drag factor, press the ready and rest buttons together and then row for a few strokes.

PM3

The PM3 is a more advanced performance monitor and is probably one of the most commonly used. The quick way of starting up the PM3 is to press the menu back button and then take a stroke or insert a log card, which is used to analyse and store any workouts so the information can be transferred to a PC. The PM3 automatically turns off after four minutes of inactivity. It is important to note that the first time the PM3 is switched on you will have to set the language, date and time. This is essential if the performance monitor is to store all your results and workouts correctly.

Main Monitor Buttons and their Functions

Change Units. This button allows the user to select one of four different units to display the results: metres (or time), calories, watts and pace/500m. It can be used in rowing displays, result screens and when setting the pace-boat.

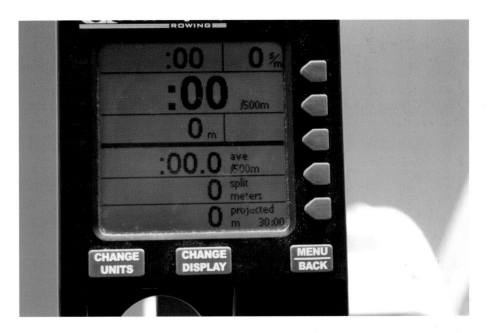

This page and pages 16–17: Five choices for the PM3 display.

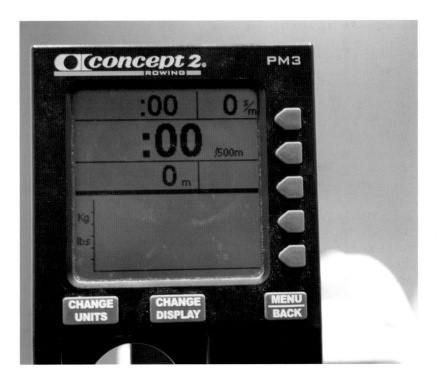

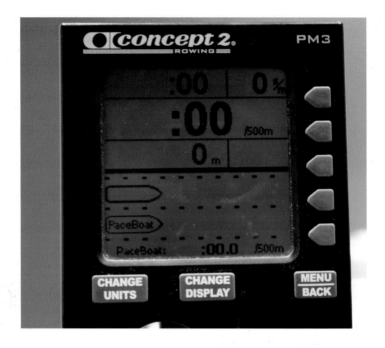

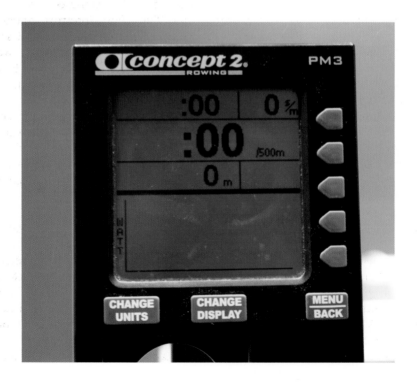

Change Display. This allows the user to select from one of five different workout displays: all data section, force curve section, pace-boat section, bar chart section and large print section. The button can only be used in the rowing displays.

Menu Back. This button returns the display to the previous screen. If the user is currently working on the main rowing display, the menu back button will end the workout and the screen turns back to the main menu.

Screen Buttons and their Functions

Just Row. This button allows the user to row up to a maximum of 50,000m without having to press any other buttons, saving all workouts longer than one minute.

Select Workout. This button provides access to five different sections: standard list, custom list, re-row, new workout and favourites.

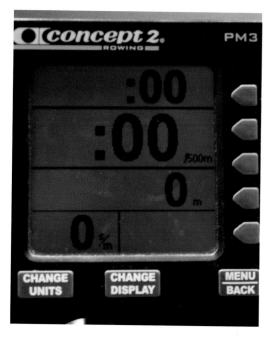

- Standard list. This section allows the user to select one of five preset workouts on the performance monitor. These cannot be changed.
- Custom list. This section includes five different workouts, each of which can be changed by different workouts that have been saved on a log card.
- Re-row. This allows the result from a previous workout to be selected as a pace-boat time.
- New workout. This section is broken down even further into five more options: single distance, single time, distance intervals, time intervals and variable intervals.
(i) The single distance option allows you to program a distance from 100m to 50,000m.
(ii) The single time option allows you to program a time from 20 seconds to 9 minutes 59 seconds.
(iii) The distance intervals option allows you to work continually from 100m to 9,999m, with rest times permitted up to 9 minutes 55 seconds.
(iv) The time intervals option allows you to work continually from 20 seconds to 59 minutes 59 seconds, with rest times up to 9 minutes 55 seconds.
(v) The variable intervals option allows the user to combine both distance (100–999,999m) and time (20 seconds–99 minutes 59 seconds). Rest times up to 9 minutes 55 seconds are allowed.
- Favourites. The favourites section stores up to five workouts per log card and is limited to thirty intervals.

Memory/Log Card. If no log card is present, the user is able to review the ten most recent workout results by date, with the oldest workout on the list automatically deleted each time. If there is a log card present, however, up to 300 workouts can be stored. The memory/log card button is broken up into five different sections: summary, monthly totals, list by date, list by type and log card utilities.

- Summary. This lists the total, and average, results recorded on a log card.
- Monthly totals. This shows a table of monthly workout totals.
- List by date. This looks up any past workout results by date.
- List by type. Allows the user to look up past workout results by type.
- Log card utilities. This section is broken down into five further options: add user, edit user, delete user, delete workout and copy workout. (i) Add user option: details of up to five users may be stored on a single log card. (ii) Edit user option: edits the name and the lifetime metres. (iii) Delete user option: deletes a name, as well as results. (iv) Delete workout option: deletes the workout results from the log card. (v) Copy workout option: copies a selected workout form the PM3 computer memory to the log card.

Information. The information button gives access to five different sections: overview, using the monitor, how to row, drag factor and replacing the battery.

- Overview.
- Using the monitor. Describes the PM3 buttons, rowing displays, workouts, as well as the log card facility.
- How to row. Provides a brief description of rowing technique.
- Drag factor. This section describes the drag factor and how the PM3 recalculates the indoor rowing machine's drag factor with every stroke, depending on the damper level setting.
- Replacing the battery. Describes the best way to replace the batteries without losing information (switch off the monitor and replace them within 5 minutes of removal).

More Options. The more options button gives access to three sections: display drag factor, utilities and edit custom list.

- Display drag factor. Allows the user to view and set the drag factor before starting the workout.
- Utilities. This section gives access to five more options: set date and time, set language, LCD contrast, battery and product ID.(i) The set date and time option is important if the user wants to store their results accurately. (ii) The set language option sets the preferred language. (iii) The LCD contrast option adjusts the contrast of the monitor. (iv) The battery option shows the percentage of battery life remaining on the performance monitor. (v) The product ID option holds all the information required for product identification.
- Edit custom list. This section allows the user to copy workouts from their favourites to the custom list if a log card is present.

PM4

The PM4 is the latest model in the performance monitor series. The basics of the monitor, including all the functions and options, are very similar to those on the PM3 model, but it has one excellent extra function, Racing. When the racing option is selected, it is possible to set up indoor races for up to eight PM4-equipped rowing machines. This can be done either wirelessly or by using Ethernet patch cables. One person creates the race on their PM4 menu and the others then log on. For a successful race, one line of indoor rowing machines should face the other line, making sure that the maximum distance between each machine on either corner is 3.35m. The individual who initially created the race will always be in lane one and can start the race once the other competitors are ready.

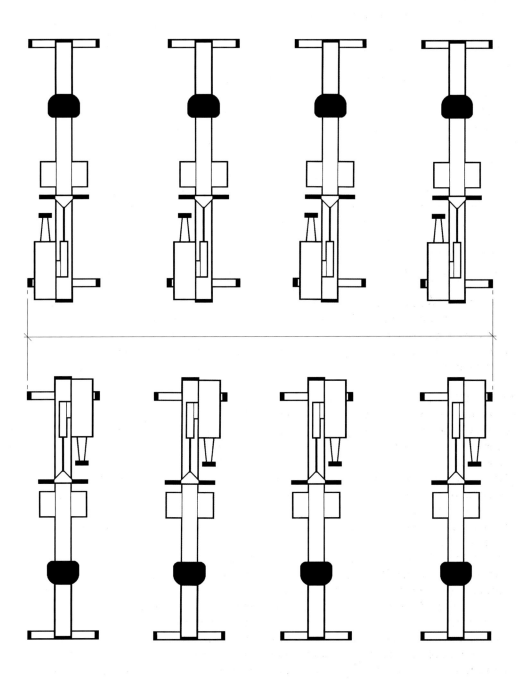

The best indoor rowing machine racing layout for PM4 machines.

3 Indoor Rowing Technique and Common Mistakes

Perfect Practice Makes Perfect Technique

When it comes to the sport of indoor rowing, good technique is essential if you want to cover the distance in the quickest, most energy-efficient way. It is interesting to note that many of the best rowers in the world do not always have the best technique, sometimes over-compensating in different areas of the rowing stroke to allow them to cover the distance in a quick time. If, however, you want to cover the distance in the most efficient way possible and want to stay safe, it is crucial to learn good technique, especially if you are only starting out in the sport.

Learn Something New
When our bodies learn something new, the process can be broken down into two different stages: the learning phase and the automatic phase. The learning phase is when electrical impulses are sent through the nervous system from the brain. For indoor rowing, our mind and body slowly break down each section of the rowing stroke at a slow pace: as the body gets used to the load, range and speed of the stroke, the pace of the stroke will increase and allow the body to work out how the stroke relates to the movement of other muscles in the body. The automatic phase is entered when the body automatically knows everything about the indoor rowing stroke – what to do and when to do it.

When you are in the automatic phase of learning, you no longer have to think about every detail of what you are doing on an indoor rowing machine.

Technique

The following technique is based on safe and effective principles of body biomechanics. It will allow your indoor rowing stroke to be as efficient as possible, as well as helping to reduce any risk of injury. Different body types, builds and muscular imbalances require variations of the indoor rowing stroke, but the ideal rowing stoke can be shown in five different phases: the start position, the leg drive, the arm pull, the release and the finish position.

Start Position
When you are in the start position you need to make sure your shins are close to vertical, with your chest high. Your arms should be straight out in front of your body and relaxed.

Leg Drive
During the leg drive phase, both your legs should push down into the footplates of the indoor rowing machine as your body begins to move backwards. Throughout the leg drive phase of the indoor rowing stroke, you should always make sure that both your arms remain straight throughout the movement.

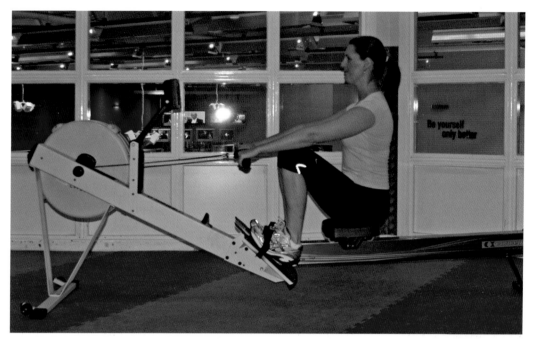

Remember to have vertical shins in the start position.

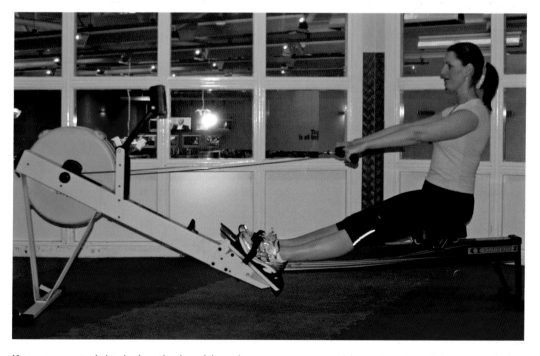

Keep arms straight during the leg drive phase.

Arm Pull

During the arm pull phase, your body should have stopped moving backwards. You then pull both your arms and the handle past the knees and strongly into your body. Throughout the arm pull phase, your legs should remain flat and both forearms should be horizontal throughout the movement.

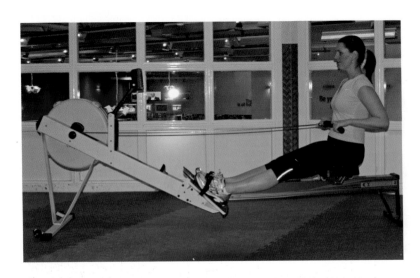

Pull the handle strongly into the body for the arm pull phase.

The Release

When you reach the release phase of the stroke, release both arms back out in front of your body to a fully extended position, remembering to keep your arms relaxed. As your body rocks forward from your hips, slide your whole body forward again, making sure to maintain good arm and body position.

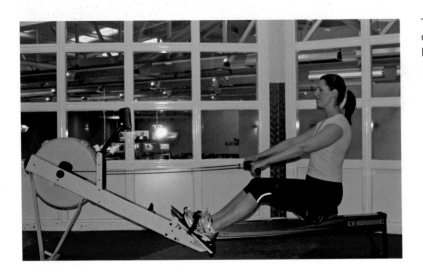

Try to stay relaxed during the release phase.

Finish Position

When the indoor rowing stroke is finished, your position should be the same as when you started. Both your shins are close to vertical and your chest remains high. Your arms are straight and relaxed. From this position you are ready to start the next stroke and repeat.

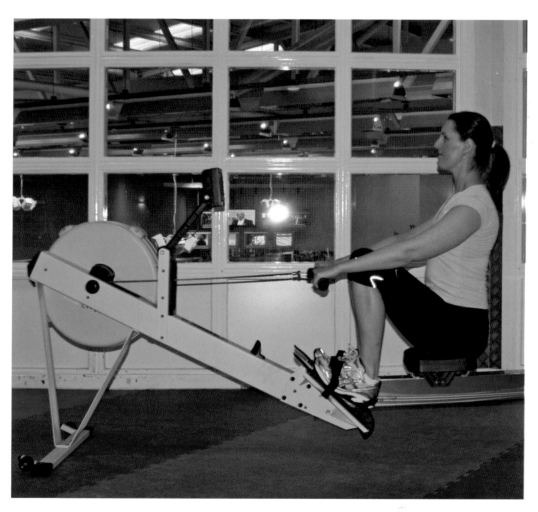

Keep the chest high for the finish position.

Common Technique Faults

As with any sport, there are certain common technique faults that many individuals taking part in indoor rowing will encounter, hindering your performance and perhaps even leading to injury.

Bent Arms
This problem arises when the individual starts the leg drive phase of the stroke by pulling with their arms, rather than pushing with both legs. When your arms are bent, the arm muscles and those connected to the arms remain tight and contracted. This constant state of tension will lead to an increase in what is known as muscle lactic acid, a by-product of exercise that can result in early fatigue and destroy your exercise performance. The solution is to start the drive phase of the indoor rowing stroke by pushing with both legs, always keeping your arms straight and relaxed.

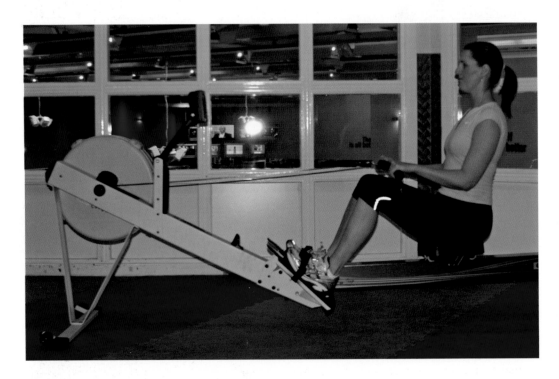

Rowing with bent arms will result in early fatigue.

High Pull
The high pull occurs when a user pulls the indoor rowing machine's bar too high towards the end of the rowing stroke, allowing their back to lean too far back. This increases the amount of energy used to swing the body back through the upright position, resulting in early fatigue during the workout. The solution is to draw the handle into the body, keeping the wrists and forearms straight, remembering to slide both elbows past your body throughout the rowing stroke.

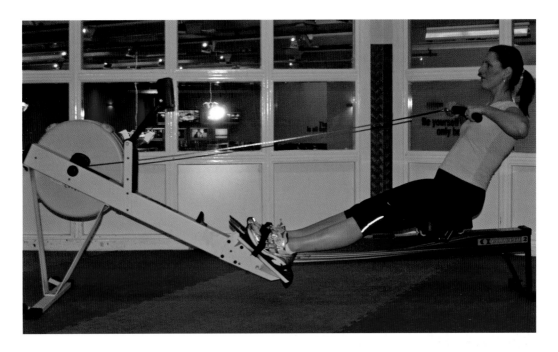

Too much energy is used if you pull the handle too high.

Bent Wrists

Bent wrists is a fault that can be spotted throughout the different sections of the indoor rowing stroke. If you row with bent wrists throughout the stroke, there is an increased risk of getting an injury. The stroke can be carried out far more efficiently when the resistance created can pass through the centre of all joints. The only solution here is to have regular checks when you are rowing to make sure the wrists remain straight and flat through each stage of the stroke.

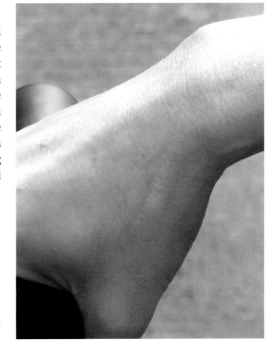

Rowing with bent wrists can increase the risk of injury.

Bending Your Back Too Early

This fault arises when the individual starts to lean back and swing their body, instead of driving back with the legs and keeping their back straight. Leaning back too early in the drive phase of the rowing stroke results in a weaker stroke. The solution is to always drive back with your legs first; only after that should you then tip back slightly with arms extended, before pullimg the handle in.

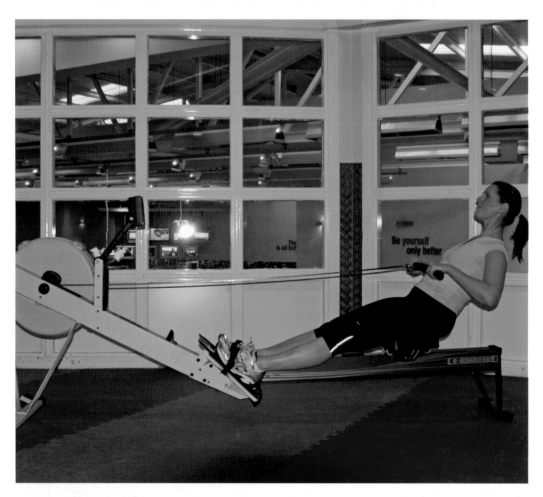

Bending backwards too early will result in a weaker stroke.

Over-reaching Back

This occurs during the release phase of the indoor rowing stroke, when an individual stretches too far forward, tipping their head forward in the process and reaching in towards the flywheel. If you find yourself in this position, you will have to start the drive phase of your next stroke in a weaker position, pulling with a heavy load and risking injury. The solution to check that your chest remains high on the way back in, remembering to keep your body tilted slightly forward.

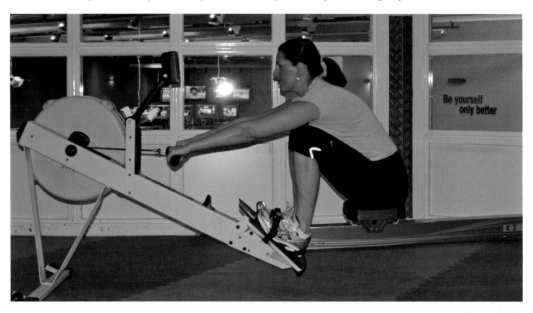

Over-reaching will affect the next stroke.

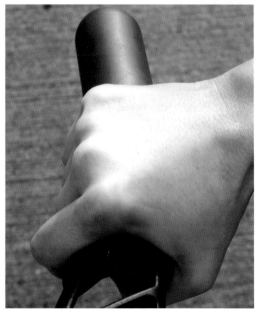

Gripping Too Tightly

Gripping an indoor rowing machine's handle too tightly throughout every phase of the rowing stroke will result in your shoulders becoming hunched, leading to early fatigue in your upper body during the movement. The solution is loosen up your grip, especially on the way back in from your rowing stroke.

Gripping the handle too tightly wastes energy quickly.

4 Goal Setting and Motivation

Setting Goals

Setting yourself fitness-based goals is one of the most important things you can do if you want to get ahead and accomplish more than you ever thought possible. Many individuals give up their fitness regime early because they lack a goal and have no firm direction as to where they want to go with their workout routine. Before embarking on any health and fitness routine, it is essential to set clear and realistic goals. The popular goal of 'I want to lose a little weight' might be effective in the short term, but the reality is that, if you want to see success in the long term, you need to be a lot more specific with what it is you want and when you want it to happen.

One of the first things you need to consider when setting fitness goals is to think back to past exercise plans you have followed and ask yourself why you gave them up. Identify what it was that scuppered your good intentions previously, so you do not repeat the same mistakes during your indoor rowing fitness routine. Many people believe that it is too difficult to fit regular fitness into their busy lifestyles, but if you want it enough, you will make time for it. It is important to find a balance between your indoor rowing routines, work life and home life. Treat your fitness goal as you would any other work or family project, devoting the appropriate time you feel it needs to be successful.

Long-term Goals

A good piece of advice to get you started is to buy a notebook or diary and write down your

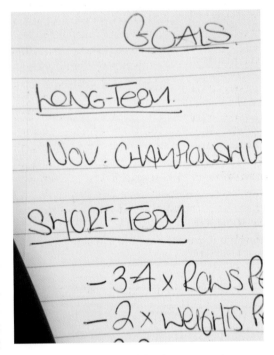

Write down your goals for better results.

goal for the future. Ideally you should try to choose one that can be achieved within three to six months. Many individuals who set their goals longer than that tend to lose interest somewhere down the line and quit early. Poor goal setting will lead to nothing but disappointment, so be realistic with what is possible: do not have a goal to row 2000m in 6 minutes 30 seconds within three months, for example, if your best time to date is 11 minutes. Your long-term goal should be a clear target for you to aim towards. It is crucial to commit yourself to this goal and treat it as if it is the most important project you have ever set yourself. If you do not take goals seriously then you will start to make excuses at some point and your chances of success will be greatly reduced.

Short-term Goals

Short-term goals will keep you motivated week-to-week and day-to-day. In your diary, or notebook, you should write down weekly and daily targets that can be ticked off as and when they are completed. Short-term goals can include such factors as rest times, nutrition and workout sessions. They should be as clear as possible: for example, you might want to set yourself a target to drink more water, eat more fruit, lift heavier weights, increase your rowing distance or decrease your rowing time. The important thing to remember is to keep every target, no matter how small, as specific as possible and read them daily to keep them fresh in your mind. Short-term goals will help you reach those long-term goals, so treat them seriously.

SMART Goals

To maximize performance and get your health and body shape to the way you want it to be, it is important to plan and follow SMART goals.

Specific

Each goal you think of should be as specific as possible, so that you know exactly what to do and when to do it, in order to reach your ultimate fitness goal. Too many individuals end up being too vague with what they want out of their fitness routines. If your goal is to lose weight, then break it up into exactly how much it is you want to lose and when you want to lose it by; if your goal is to improve your fitness, then take a fitness test to find out your starting point. You should plan training sessions to achieve exact times, distances and levels, maybe even setting

S	specific
M	measurable
A	aggressive
R	relevant
T	time-related

yourself the target of competing in a future indoor rowing event or competition.

Measurable

Measuring your progress towards any goal is essential to allow you to see whether or not your plan is actual working. If you do not measure your progress you will never know whether you need to scrap your current workout routine and try a different strategy to keep you on track to reach your goal. Measurable goals will also help you continue a steady progress throughout each short-term goal, so helping to prevent a minor setback turning into a major failure as you progress towards your ultimate long-term goal.

Aggressive

People who set goals at the upper end of their ability tend to do far better than individuals who set themselves easy goals they know they can accomplish. Making your goals more aggressive will not only inspire you to put more effort into each training session on the indoor rowing machine, but you will also gain a fantastic sense of achievement when you accomplish them.

Relevant

When planning your short-term goals, it is important to make sure they are relevant to the final long-term goal you have chosen. For example, if you have a long-term goal to complete a marathon on the indoor rowing machine in six months time, should you plan four sessions a week on the bike and only one short session on the indoor rowing machine? No. Every short-term goal you set should be another step towards your final goal.

Time-related

All your goals should be realistic within the time available. If your goal is to lose three stone in weight, for example, do not expect to drop all the weight in a couple of weeks. Believing unrealistic time frames for your goals will only leave you disheartened and annoyed when you do not reach them. All you have to do to reach the goal is to break it down into more manageable chunks. So, instead of three stones in such a short period, give yourself more time to get there and aim to lose only two to three pounds a week. That way you will stay motivated as you achieve each of the smaller, more manageable, weight losses each week.

Motivation

Stay Positive

Successful people who reach every goal they set themselves possess certain person-ality factors that set them apart from others who give up early and do not get what they want. This is the same for all types of goal-setting, including health and fitness. Individuals who reach every goal they set themselves will have vision, a plan, belief and determination.

To be successful, you need to be certain about what you want to achieve and you should always see the light at the end of the tunnel. Such people always work out their real objectives and have a vision as to where they are going and what the result will be. To turn that vision into a reality, you need to have a plan that will channel all of your efforts effectively, boosting motivation and resulting in better performances. Self-belief is one of the most powerful predictors to success. A strong belief that you will be successful will not only knock back any negativity you have, but it will also make you work harder in every workout session and more happy with what you are doing, helping you to achieve more and handle any failure better. Finally, determination is imperative if you want to reach any health and fitness goals you set yourself. Too many people give up early because they give up on themselves. Someone who is determined will keep moving forward, not bothered by any setbacks they meet on the way. They have only one thing in their mind – their personal fitness goal.

Barriers

Starting out is always tough and no one is perfect. When it comes to fitness everyone will have a moment of weakness and the excuses will always be the same – 'I'll do more tomorrow', 'I don't have the time'. The list can be endless.

If you notice that you are constantly making excuses before you reach even your short-term goal, the chances of making your long-term goal are going to be slim. Sticking to your training programme can take a lot of commitment and sometimes a situation arises that is out of your control, making you move away from your fitness routine. The trick is to ensure that any variation from your fitness routines is only temporary. You have to get the balance right with your life and training. Too much of anything can be bad for you, so be firm with yourself. Minor setbacks will always appear, but you have to overcome these barriers if you want to be successful. You should always expect the unexpected. The following list includes some of the more common barriers that can get in the way of your fitness routine and stop you getting the results you deserve.

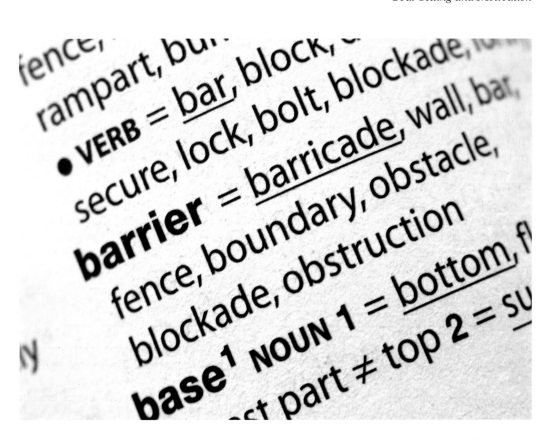

Learn to overcome any barriers that will slow down your progress.

Barrier: Work
Solution: If you are one of the unfortunate people who work long hours and do not think you have time to train, then think again. Why not try to get up earlier and train before work or head to the gym for lunch for a quick blast on the indoor rowing machine. It is not necessary to spend long hours on the machine in order to get any benefit. Once you turn your exercise routines into a habit, you will be amazed how it will be difficult to break.

Barrier: Family commitments
Solution: If you feel that family commitments will upset your fitness routine, then talk to your family and let them know what you are doing and, more importantly, why you want to do it. Once your new health and fitness lifestyle has your family's supports, they will be more understanding of other fitness-related commitments you may have down the line.

Barrier: Lack of motivation
Solution: One of the most commonest reasons people give for leaving gyms is that they lack motivation, despite the fantastic range of facilities that gyms have to offer. To rekindle your enthusiasm for training, why not train with a friend, hire a personal trainer, or even set your sights on a specific indoor rowing event in the future.

Barrier: Don't have the energy
Solution: Many people believe that they do not have the energy to work out. The reason

you do not have the energy is because you do not do any form of fitness training. Good nutrition and the right amount of exercise on an indoor rowing machine will increase your energy levels.

Barrier: Don't have the time
Solution: By far the most common excuse that people give for not taking up a fitter lifestyle is that they just do not have the time to exercise. If you really want to reach your fitness goal and change your lifestyle for the better, you will make fitness a priority. The recommended activity for an adult to improve their health is thirty minutes a day for five days a week, making a total of two-and-a-half hours each week. There are 168 hours in a week – still think you cannot find the time?

Barrier: Transport
Solution: Some people live far away from their nearest gym and find it difficult to travel, but what if you work in a city? Chances are there will be a gym somewhere in any sizeable city or town. Why not pack your training bag and train before work, during your lunchtime or straight after work before you head back home. You could even cycle to and from work if the journey is practicable – every little bit helps. You could also train outside near where you live or, if you would rather train in the comfort of your own home, why not purchase an indoor rowing machine. There are always options to get fit and healthy if you really want to.

Barrier: Health problems
Solution: Some individuals would love to start an exercise programme but feel they cannot because of underlying health issues. One massive positive of exercise is that it will help alleviate many health problems, including diabetes, osteoporosis, heart disease, arthritis, cholesterol, depression, blood pressure, a weakened immune system, obesity and even cancer. If you are careful about what you do and seek out professional advice, you can do an effective fitness programme with confidence, especially on an indoor rowing machine, due to the low impact nature of the sport.

Barrier: Injury
Solution: Depending on the severity of the injury, there is a good chance you could still find something to do to make sure you do not lose your fitness or strength. The best way is to seek advice from a local fitness or health professional regarding suggestions as to what you can still do if you want to continue some form of fitness training. Do not let injuries put a stop to your ambitions.

Barrier: Too expensive
Solution: Money is always a worry, but as the number of budget gyms steadily increases, the overall cost of using top of the range equipment, and seeking advice from a qualified fitness team, is relatively small. If you feel that gyms are not for you, or that you prefer to have a small gym at home, you can always seek out older ranges or second-hand indoor rowing machines on the internet. You may be amazed at how little equipment you actually need to get the results you want – you do not have to break the bank.

Barrier: Going on holiday
Solution: It is hard to believe, but some people see going on holiday as a barrier. Such an occasion should be a well-deserved break and reward. You should use that time to recharge your batteries. If you find going on holiday more of a worry, though, keep in mind the opportunities you can take to maintain your fitness: the pool, outdoor walks, hiring a bicycle, body weight exercises in your hotel room … the list goes on. You might not be able to do your usual routine, especially if the hotel does not have a gym, but it is good to mix things up and try something different – your body will love the benefits.

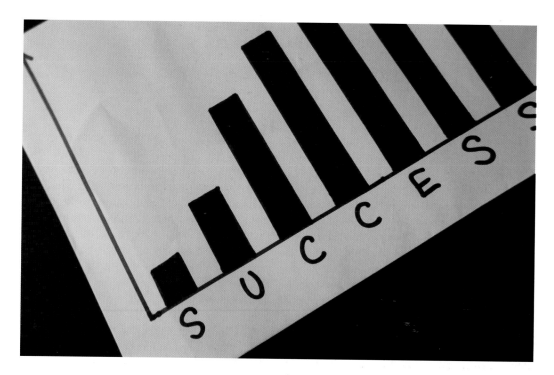

The right support and environment will lead to success.

Tips for Success

Friends and Family

You will improve your chances of success if you can get the support of at least one person close to you, someone who understands your motives for what you are doing. Have a chat with the person you feel would be the most supportive and talk through everything that you want to do. You may be amazed at the effect another's positive attitude will have on you, especially when you know they will be there to keep pushing you in the right direction if you ever find the going gets tough.

Motivating Surroundings

Fitness training should give you a high, leaving you feeling good about yourself; if you hate it, you can guarantee that you will not stick to it. Try to create a motivating environment that works for you. For some people that might mean being a member of a certain gym or joining in with a specialized club; for others it could mean listening to certain music while training or even enlisting the help of a training buddy. Knowing you are both there for each other, pushing one other in the workout, is always a good thing. Remember, everyone is different, so consider what would work for you; it will help you train harder and get results quicker.

Reward Yourself

A small reward every time you reach a new fitness goal is an excellent way to keep you on track and boost your motivation. The reward could be as simple as a gold star in your training diary or, if you prefer, you could book a full-body massage to help your body recover.

5   The Start and End of Every Workout

Warm-Up

Warming up your body before any form of exercise is essential if you want to make sure you get a safe and effective workout. The warm-up will have three main benefits: it will increase your heart and respiratory rate; it will raise your body temperature; and it will even help prepare you mentally for your indoor rowing workout ahead. It takes time for a body to change from its normal state to the point where it is ready to perform vigorous exercise. If the heart rate is not increased gradually, it can result in an irregular heartbeat, which can be very dangerous for a less active, or older, person. A good warm-up will switch on the body's aerobic system (performing with oxygen) and allow the body to reach a steady state. Without a warm-up, our body will provide anaerobic energy (performing without oxygen), which can lead to the formation of a waste product in the muscles known as lactic acid.

The main reasons why you should always warm up before an indoor rowing session are to increase the blood flow to the muscles, the rate of muscle contraction (as well as the efficiency of opposite working muscles), the metabolic rate, tissue flexibility and your mental awareness. A proper warm-up, depending on the intensity of your indoor rowing session, can require between five and twenty minutes (for recommended warm-up times for different rowing sessions, see the table later in this chapter). Warm-ups can be divided into two main categories: general and specific.

General. A general warm-up can be a low-intensity exercise or series of movements that do not necessarily have to relate to indoor rowing. There are many variations of this type of warm-up, for example, warming up on a stationary bike before starting to do a weights session, or warming up on an X-trainer machine before starting an indoor rowing workout.

Specific. A specific warm-up is still low intensity, but the difference is that the moves will mimic closely the moves you are about to do in your main workout, for example, doing body weight lunges and press-ups before a weights workout, or a short, low-intensity stint on an indoor rowing machine before starting the main indoor rowing workout.

There has always been speculation as to whether a warm-up actually benefits your performance and if it really can help to prevent injuries. Unfortunately, for every researcher who states that warm-ups are essential, there are just as many who claim there is no benefit to warming up. This can be very confusing for someone who is just starting on a new health and fitness lifestyle, but the fact is that your body will move more effectively and efficiently after a proper warm-up, owing to the benefits mentioned earlier. It might not guarantee that you stay injury-free, but it will enhance your workout performance. Considering a warm-up can take as little as five minutes, I would recommend an easy intensity warm-up before every session you undertake on an indoor rowing machine.

Cool-Down

The purpose of a cool-down is to get your body back to a steady state and help you to recover. A proper cool-down, depending on the intensity of your session, can last between five and fifteen minutes (for recommended cool-down times for different rowing sessions, see the table later in this chapter). A cool-down will have the following effects: remove the lactic acid from your muscles; minimize the muscle soreness that many people experience during the days after an indoor rowing workout; and it will help prevent blood pooling in the muscles, which can lead to dizziness. Getting into the habit of doing cool-downs after every indoor rowing workout can take a lot of discipline, but if you want to get the most out of your next session, then remember to do a good cool-down to reduce the effect of delayed onset muscle soreness (DOMS), which is usually felt two days after exercise.

Warm-Up and Cooling Down on the Indoor Rowing Machine

Depending on the indoor rowing session that you are about to do, your warm-up and cool-down time can vary. For a long, low-intensity session on an indoor rowing machine you should not need as long as if you are planning to do high-intensity anaerobic sprints.

	Warm-Up	Cool-Down
Low-Intensity Aerobic Session	5–10 minutes	5–10 minutes
Medium-Intensity Interval Session	10–12 minutes	10–12 minutes
High-Intensity Interval Session	15–20 minutes	15–20 minutes

Stretches

To Stretch or not to Stretch

Muscle stretching can also be an excellent way to reduce muscle pain and aid faster recovery, although for many years it has been the subject of many debates and discussions throughout the health and fitness industry. It seems that every week there are different guidelines when it comes to stretching. Any means of improving flexibility included in a fitness programme, though, is important and should not be left out. This is especially so nowadays, when more people than ever are inactive and liable to suffer from such problems as muscular imbalances, bad posture and injury. If you can get into the habit of stretching you will find it helps not only to decrease any muscular imbalances, but it is of benefit in reducing the effects of possible joint dysfunctions and the risk of injury. To appreciate the benefits of stretching and flexibility training, it is important to understand the different types of flexibility as well as the various forms of stretching.

There are three main types of flexibility training: corrective, active and functional. Corrective flexibility is designed to improve any muscular imbalances, but it also has the effect of improving your joint range of motion; it is performed using static stretches (stretches that are held for a moderate to long time) and self-myofascial release (a self-massage technique using a foam roller).

Active flexibility is designed to improve the flexibility of your body's soft tissue by using active stretches (stretches that are held for a short time and a set number of repetitions), as well as self-myofascial release. Functional flexibility is designed to improve the flexibility of your body's soft tissue by using dynamic stretches (multi-planar stretches that move through a full range of motion). Self-myofascial release can also be used in functional flexibility.

Types of Stretching

Self-Myofascial Release
Self-myofascial release is a technique that you see used increasingly by personal trainers and gyms. Slowly roll your muscle along the foam roller, gently applying pressure. When you reach a tender part of the muscle, hold that position for approximately twenty seconds. The discomfort should ease slightly and then you continue to the next point of tension in the muscle.

Static Stretching
Static stretching is by far the most popular, and safest, form of stretching. It takes a muscle to a point of tension and holds it there for a minimum of thirty seconds. The muscle getting stretched recognizes the tension and slowly allows the muscle to relax, which then allows the individual to take the stretch a little further.

Active Stretching
Active stretching uses opposite muscles to work with each other, so that while one muscle is tensed, the other muscle is relaxed. This form of stretching is usually held for short periods of time and repeated. Most active stretches are held for approximately five seconds and repeated up to ten times. This form of stretching is popular as part of a muscle imbalance correction programme.

Dynamic Stretching
Dynamic stretching uses force and momentum to take a joint through its full range of motion. This form of stretching is popular with individuals as part of a specific sport warm-up and can be repeated up to ten times. The advantage of dynamic stretching is the timing and skill required to control and move the stretch safely.

Stretching Exercises
The following flexibility exercises are divided up according to body part, indicating the appropriate options for that muscle. Different options for the same muscle will stress the body in slightly different ways, so try each exercise listed for the body part to see what works best for you. The list of stretches is all relative to the muscles used in the rowing movement and related resistance exercises. You do not need to do every single stretch in your workout, but you should try to create your own flexibility routine, picking the stretches that you enjoy and work best where you feel tight.

Calves

Self-myofascial release:
- Place the foam roller under your calf at either the bottom or the top of the muscle.
- If you want more intensity, cross over your legs to increase the pressure on the calf.
- Draw in your abs and lift your hips, supporting your body weight with both hands.
- Slowly walk both hands, rolling your calf along the foam roller (approximately 2cm per second) to find any tender areas of the calf muscle.
- When you find a tender area, hold that position until the discomfort slowly vanishes. If the tender area does not ease after around twenty seconds you should move on to the next tender spot and repeat.

Cross over both legs to increase the intensity.

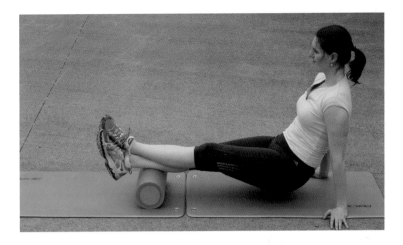

• Work your way along the whole of the calf muscle.

Static standing:
• Stand facing a wall.
• With both toes facing straight ahead, lean your upper body against the wall, keeping your back leg outstretched.
• Draw in your abs.

• Lean the pelvis and chest in towards the wall.
• Stop when you feel the point of tension in the calf muscle and hold it for approximately thirty seconds.
• (For a lower calf stretch, bend your back knee slightly, still remembering to lean in and push the back heel to the ground.)

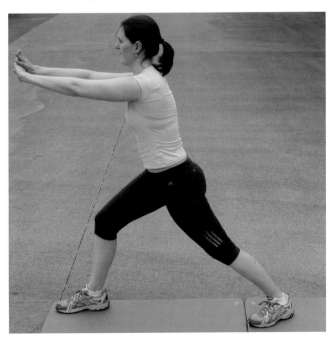

Once you feel the point of tension, hold the stretch.

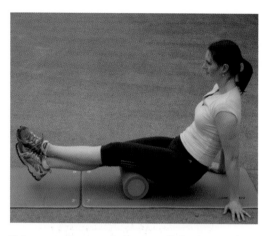

Take your time and slowly roll the hamstring over the roller.

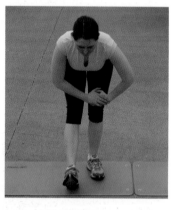

Keep the shoulders square as you lean forwards over the thigh.

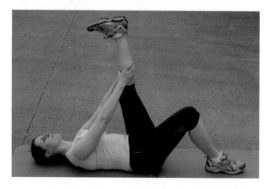

Try to keep the leg as straight as possible as you bring it back.

Hamstrings

Self-myofascial release
• Place the foam roller under your thigh at either the bottom or the top of the hamstring muscle.
• If you want more intensity, cross over your legs to increase the pressure on the muscle.
• Draw in your abs and lift your hips, supporting your body weight with both hands.
• Start to shuffle both hands, rolling the hamstring along the foam roller (approximately 2cm per second) to find any tender areas of the hamstring muscle.
• When you find a tender area, hold it until the discomfort slowly vanishes. If the tender area does not ease after twenty seconds you should then move on to the next tender spot along the muscle and repeat the hold again.
• Slowly continue your way along the whole hamstring muscle.

Static standing:
• Stand upright with your abs drawn in.
• Place one leg on a slightly raised support and slowly lean forward from the hip until you feel the point of tension. Hold for approximately thirty seconds.
• If you do not have a raised surface to rest your leg on, then you can place the leg on the ground. From here you sit back and lean forward over the leg you want to stretch, remembering to keep the front leg straight.

Static supine:
• Lying on the floor, bring one leg in towards you, holding on to the thigh.
• Draw your abs in and keep your hips flat on the ground.
• Slowly straighten out the leg you want to stretch, pressing the heel up towards the ceiling until you feel the point of tension. Hold for approximately thirty seconds.

Quadriceps

Self-myofascial release
• Place the foam roller under the front of your thigh, starting at either the bottom or the top.
• If you want more intensity, cross over your legs to increase the pressure.
• Draw in your abs and support yourself on your forearms.
• Slowly roll your quadricep along the roller (approximately 2cm per second) to find any tender areas of the muscle.
• When you find a tender area, hold it until the discomfort slowly vanishes. If the tender area does not ease after twenty seconds, move on to the next tender spot and hold again.
• Work your way along the whole muscle.

Static standing:
• Standing upright and maintaining balance, reach back and grab the front of one foot.
• Slowly bring the foot towards your buttocks, remembering to keep both knees together.
• If you want more intensity, press your foot into your hand as you pull it up.
• When you find the point of tension, hold it for approximately thirty seconds.

Static prone:
• Lying flat on your stomach, draw in your abs.
• Reach back and grab one foot.
• Slowly pull the foot towards your buttocks, remembering to keep both knees together.
• If you want more intensity, press the foot into your hand as you pull it up.
• When you find the point of tension, hold the stretch for approximately thirty seconds.

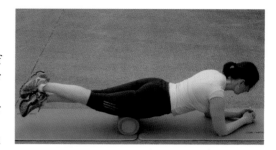

Keep your weight on your forearms as you move along the roller.

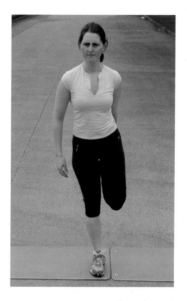

Press your foot into your hand as you bring it back to your buttocks.

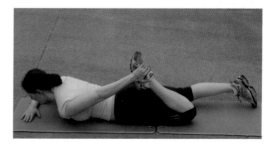

Try to keep your knees close together throughout the stretch.

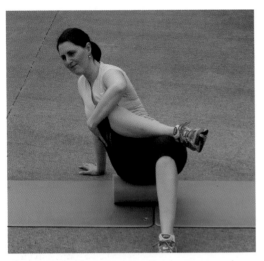

Pull the knee in towards your body for more intensity.

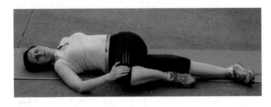

Try to keep both shoulders down on the floor for a better stretch.

Back (Latissimus Dorsi)

Self-myofascial release:
• Place the foam roller under the area of your armpit, lying on your side with the arm nearer the floor outstretched in front.
• Draw in your abs.

Glutes

Self-myofascial release:
• Sit on top of the foam roller, positioning yourself on the back of your hip.
• Cross one foot onto the opposite knee.
• Draw in your abs and support yourself with one hand behind you. Use the other hand to pull the knee towards your body.
• Slowly roll along the roller (2cm per second) to find any tender areas of the muscle.
• When you find a tender area, hold it until the discomfort slowly vanishes. If the tender area does not ease after twenty seconds, move on to the next tender spot and hold again.
• Work your way along the muscle area.

Static supine:
• Lying flat on your back, cross one leg over the other.
• Draw in your abs.
• With one hand on the outside of your thigh, slowly pull towards your opposite shoulder until the point of tension is found, then hold for approximately thirty seconds.

• Slowly roll back and forward along the roller (approximately 2cm per second) to find any tender areas of the muscle.
• When you find a tender area, hold it until the discomfort slowly vanishes. If the tender area does not ease after twenty seconds, move on to the next tender spot and hold again.

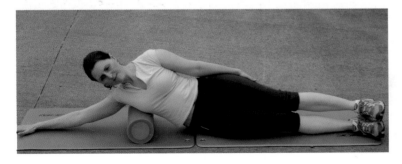

Roll only a small area just under the armpit for the best results.

Static kneeling:
- Start by kneeling on the ground and place one arm outstretched in front of you on the ground, remembering to keep your thumb pointed upwards.

- Draw in your abs.
- Slowly sit your weight back until you feel the point of tension and hold for approximately thirty seconds.

Sit your weight back towards your heels as you press the arm down.

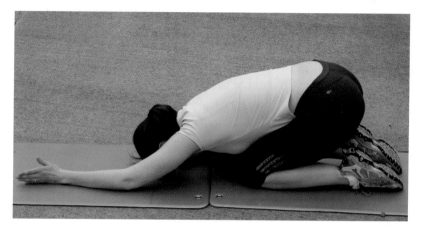

Back (Erector Spinae)

Self-myofascial release:
- Place the foam roller under your back.
- Cross your arms to the opposite shoulder and lie back on the roller so that it is positioned on the upper back.
- Draw in your abs and raise your hips.

- Slowly roll back and forward along the roller (approximately 2cm per second) to find any tender areas of the muscle.
- When you find a tender area, hold it until the discomfort slowly vanishes. If the tender area does not ease after twenty seconds, move on to the next tender spot and hold again.

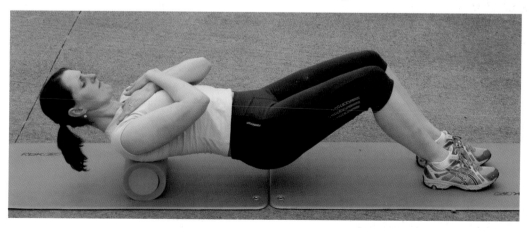

Keep both arms crossed to open up the area you want to foam roll.

Static seated:
- Sitting on the floor, bend one leg in and cross it over the other leg.
- Draw in your abs.

- Using the opposite arm to the leg that is bent, slowly push against the leg until the point of tension is found and hold for approximately thirty seconds.

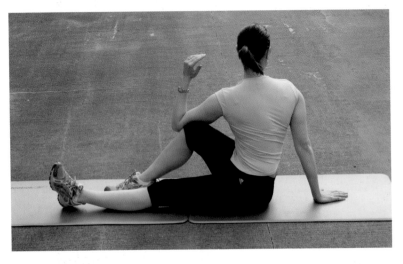

Press into the bent leg as you twist your body as far as you can.

Static supine:
- Start by lying flat on your back.
- Draw in your abs.
- Bend both knees with your feet on the ground.

- Reach out, hold on to your knees and slowly pull your thighs in towards your chest until you feel the point of tension. Hold for approximately thirty seconds.

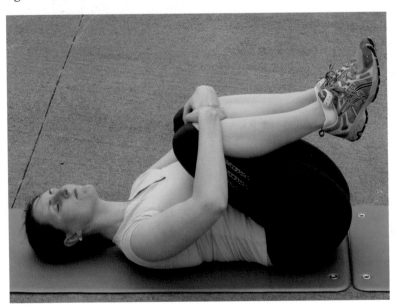

Keep the shoulders down low as you hug both knees.

Shoulders

Static standing:
- Standing upright, draw your abs in.
- Reach one arm across the front of your body, remembering to keep the shoulder position low.
- With the other arm, hook the arm and slowly pull back until you find the point of tension. Hold for approximately thirty seconds.

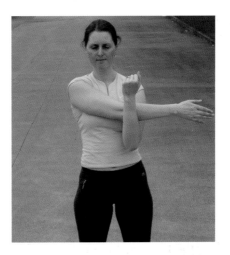

Chest

Static standing:
- Standing upright, draw in your abs.
- Place both of your palms on the small of your back.
- Slowly squeeze both elbows in close together, until you feel the point of tension. Hold for approximately thirty seconds.

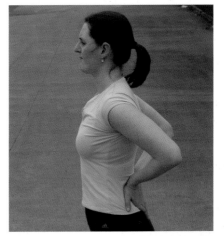

Wrist Flexors and Extensors

Static standing:
- Standing upright, make sure your abs are drawn in.
- Extend one arm out in front of your body and, with the other hand, slowly push your palm down towards the ground, keeping your fingers straight, until you feel the point of tension.

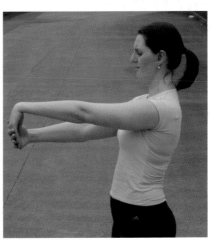

TOP: Keep the body square as you pull the arm in towards you.

MIDDLE:
The head should be high as you squeeze both elbows close.

BOTTOM:
Apply gentle pressure until you feel the point of tension.

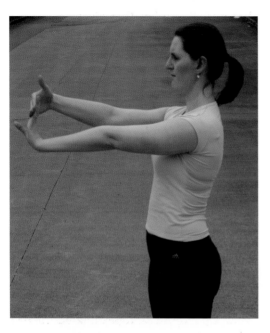

Make sure the pressure you apply is slow and controlled.

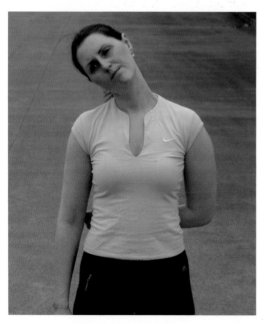

Drop the ear close to your shoulder to feel the neck stretch.

• With the same arm extended out in front, now slowly pull your palm up, keeping your fingers straight, until you feel the point of tension. Hold for approximately thirty seconds.

Neck (Flexors)

Static standing:
• Standing upright, draw your abs in.
• Place your left arm behind your body.
• Tuck your chin and slowly drop your ear to your right shoulder until you feel the point of tension. Hold for approximately thirty seconds.
• If you want more intensity, gently apply pressure to your head with your right hand.

Neck (Extensors)

Static standing:
• Standing upright, draw your abs in.
• Tuck your chin and slowly drop your head down towards your chest until you feel the point of tension. Hold for approximately thirty seconds.
• If you want more intensity, gently apply pressure to your head with your hand.

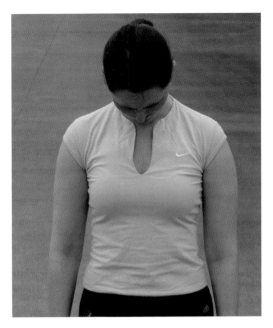

Keep the chin tucked in tightly for a good stretch.

Dynamic Stretches/Exercises

Dynamic stretching consists of simple movements that can be used as part of your warm-up. Remember that for each of the following dynamic exercises it is important to start the movement steadily, slowly building up the speed and keeping it under control at all times. All exercises are usually performed with body weight only, but if you prefer to increase the intensity, you can use a light weight or medicine ball.

Woodchop Low to High

- Start by standing upright with your feet hips-width apart.
- Holding on to a light weight or medicine ball, and keeping your abs drawn in, bend both knees and bring the weight down by your side.
- Slowly lift and rotate upwards, allowing your hips to turn and pivoting on the ball of your foot.
- Repeat for up to ten times.
- Repeat on the other side.

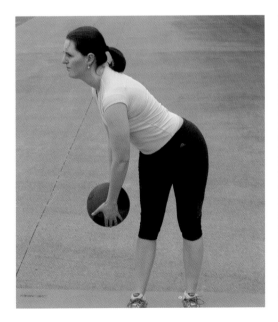

Woodchop low to high: start down low with the medicine ball and keep toes straight ahead.

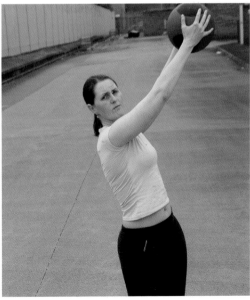

Woodchop low to high: allow your body to twist around and up high.

Pendulum
- Start by standing upright with your feet hips-width apart.
- Holding on to a light weight or medicine ball, and keeping your abs drawn in, bend both knees and bring the weight down between your legs.
- Slowly lift and extend up towards your head.
- Repeat for up to ten times.

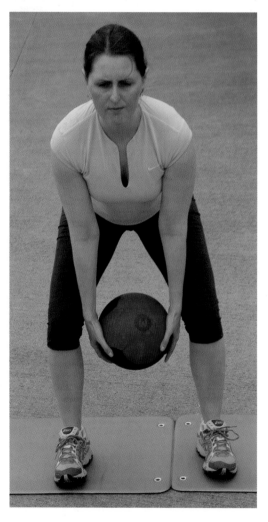

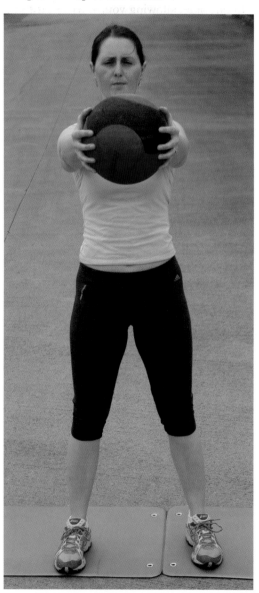

Pendulum: try to keep your head up at the bottom of the move.

Pendulum: keep the arms straight as you swing the medicine ball up.

Spinal Rotation
- Start by standing upright with your feet hips-width apart.
- Holding on to a light weight or medicine ball, and keeping your abs drawn in, rotate to one side, allowing your hips to turn and pivoting onto the ball of your foot.

- Keep both arms close to your chest throughout the move. In order to increase the intensity you can always extend both arms out for the move.
- Repeat for up to ten times, alternating each side.

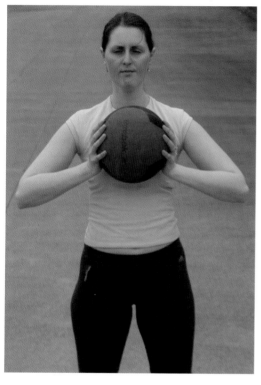

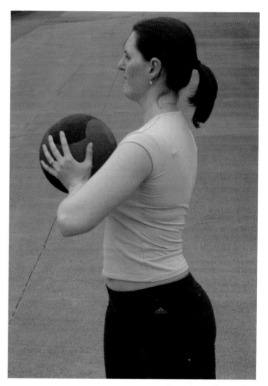

Spinal rotation: keep the medicine ball close to your chest.

Spinal rotation: the ball remains close as you rotate your upper body to the side.

Press-Up with Rotation

- Start in a press-up position, with your hands just outside shoulders-width apart.
- Draw in your abs.
- Slowly lower your body down into a press-up, keeping your body level with the floor.
- Push your body back up to the start position, then slowly rotate your body, reaching one arm up to the ceiling and return back to the start position.
- Repeat for up to ten times.
- Repeat on the other side.

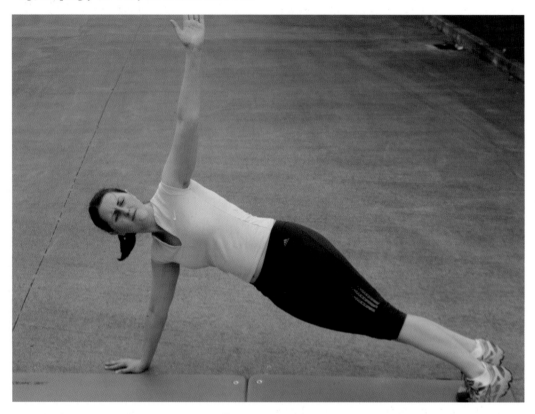

Press-up with rotation: slowly rotate and look towards the arm that is reaching high.

Cat Arch

- Start on the floor, with your hands and knees on the ground, and keeping your hands shoulders-width apart and knees hips-width apart.
- Draw in your abs.
- Slowly round your spine and tuck your rear underneath. Pause for a moment, then arch your spine and point your rear up to the ceiling.
- Get the move smooth throughout.
- Repeat for up to ten times.

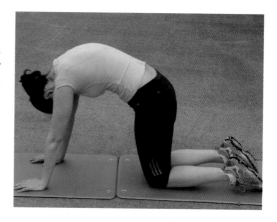

Cat arch: the chin is tightly tucked in as you round the back up high.

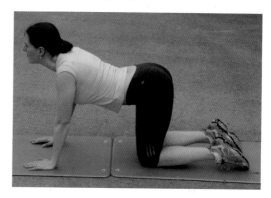

Cat arch: look up as you arch your back.

Supine Rotation

- Start by lying on the floor with your knees bent and feet lifted.
- Keep your arms relaxed and place both of them out to the side.
- Draw in your abs.
- Slowly drop your knees to one side, allowing your spine to twist with the movement.
- Rotate as low as you find to be comfortable, then return to the start position and repeat on the other side.
- Get the move smooth throughout.
- Repeat for up to ten times.

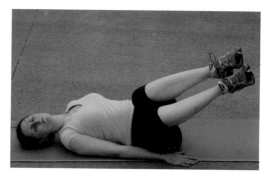

Supine rotation: don't let the shoulders lift as you rotate your lower body.

6 Benefits of Cardiovascular Training

When it comes to cardiovascular training for the heart and lungs, knowledge is power. Once you understand what it is you are doing and why you are doing it, you will not only save time, but you will also give yourself the best chance to get the results you want. To get the most out of the indoor rowing machine workouts listed in Chapter 10, it is crucial to understand the different intensities, as well as the main energy systems used by our body. There are two main energy systems: the aerobic system and the anaerobic system. The anaerobic system can be divided up into two further systems: the anaerobic lactic system and the anaerobic alactic system.

The aerobic system needs oxygen to function. It takes oxygen in, then transports and uses it. The aerobic system is used by our bodies when the exercise intensity is at an easy to moderate level and generally lasts for longer than about four minutes. Cardiovascular exercise is able to maintain this energy system intensity since it stimulates the heart and blood to deliver oxygen to the working muscles. The anaerobic lactic energy system does not need oxygen. A major by-product of this system is lactic acid. The anaerobic lactic system is generally used by our bodies only when the supply of oxygen is low and the exercise intensity is high, lasting from approximately fifteen seconds up to four minutes, depending on the individual's fitness level. The anaerobic alactic energy system also does not require oxygen, but it also does not produce lactic acid. Generally this system is only used when the exercise intensity is extremely high for a short period of time, usually under fifteen seconds.

Basic Training Concepts

When thinking about your workout plan and individual indoor rowing sessions, it is important to first go through the FIST checklist to make sure your training is progressing and that you are getting the most out of each individual indoor rowing session. The FIST checklist is as follows:

Frequency

Frequency refers to the number of training sessions, both indoor rowing sessions and resistance sessions, in a given time. Frequency can also refer to the consistency of the workouts. Remember that it is always better to get into a routine of doing shorter workouts regularly than long workouts every so often. If you get into the habit of so-called crash training, this will only result in over-training, as well as risking injury.

F	frequency
I	intensity
S	specific
T	technique

Intensity

Intensity refers to the demand that is placed on the body during the workout. To make sure you adapt to the exercise safely and effectively, the intensity should gradually be increased and never rushed. Keep in mind, though, that the intensity of your workouts should increase as your fitness improves. It is also important to always listen to your body before, during and after training. Take it easier on the days your body is tired and take advantage of the days that you are feeling good – you are only human and not a machine.

Specific

Specific refers to keeping your workouts on track for your chosen goal. Each training session, whether it is an indoor rowing workout or a resistance training workout, should be specific to your fitness or indoor rowing goal. For example, if each of your indoor rowing sessions is always no more than 1,000m, do not expect to be able to complete a marathon (42,195m) on the indoor rower in the next month.

Technique

Technique is self-explanatory. You should spend time to perfect your technique on the indoor rowing machine. Good technique will reduce the risk of injury and will make you a more efficient rower, resulting in better results.

Recovery

A balanced approach with your training routine is best, if you want your body to recover properly for the next workout session. To get the most out of your training and achieve the best results possible, recovery is a major factor. It is important to remember that training on its own will not improve your performance, but training with sufficient recovery time will boost your indoor rowing performance. If you want to improve your rowing, it is not about how much training you can do, but rather, how much training can you recover from. There are many different ways to let your body recover. The following topics cover the more popular forms of recovery. Remember, though, that each will be relative to the intensity of the previous indoor rowing or resistance workout session.

Cool-down

As described in Chapter 5, cool-downs are an excellent way to help flush away waste by-products from the muscle, such as lactic acid. The cool-down should be a very easy intensity. Always remember that the more intense your workout, the longer your cool-down should be.

Fluid and Nutrition

During an indoor rowing workout you will lose essential fluids that need to be replaced, unless you want your workout quality to suffer. You should always have a water bottle and keep yourself well hydrated before exercise, and then during and after the chosen workout session. It is also important to replenish your body with a good post-workout snack (see Chapter 13).

Sleep

Many still do not realize the importance of a good night's sleep and the benefit it can give to your indoor rowing workouts. Sleep can vary from person to person, but a good goal is to average seven to eight hours each night, if possible. It is crucial to get into a regular routine with your sleep, if you want to improve your performance. Sleep patterns that vary widely from night to night can have a negative effect on your indoor rowing sessions.

Active Rest

Active rest is probably best suited to more experienced indoor rowers or those who need to stay more active during the competition season, but who feel they need a break from using an indoor rowing machine. A good example of this is to work at a lower intensity on another piece of equipment, such as a cross trainer or bike.

Heart Rates and Intensities

Training intensities can be divided into many different categories and sub-categories, but to keep things simple it is best to concentrate on three main categories: low (aerobic), medium (threshold) and high (anaerobic) intensity. As a guide to how hard you are working and what intensity you are in, understanding heart rates is crucial. One of the best pieces of fitness equipment you can invest in is a heart rate monitor. Your heart rate gauges how hard you are working by showing how fast your heart is beating in beats per minute – the higher your heart rate, the harder you are working (the harder your heart is working to pump oxygen to the working muscles) and vice versa. When working with heart rates to work out the intensity of your indoor rowing session, one of the first things you need to do is identify your resting heart rate is, as well as your maximum heart rate. Without these two numbers, your heart rate zones can be wildly inaccurate.

Resting Heart Rate

To make sure you get a true resting heart rate, you should take it first thing in the morning when you are still lying down. The best time to take your resting heart rate is a few minutes after waking up, so make sure you plan ahead and have your heart rate monitor next to your bed from the night before. Heart rate can be affected by many different factors, so you should take into consideration whether you have a stressful day ahead, as this can easily elevate your beats per minute. The average resting heart rate for a moderately active individual is seventy-five beats per minute, but if you find that your resting heart rate is much

higher, try not to panic too much, because as your fitness improves so will your resting heart rate.

Maximum Heart Rate

There are many ways to calculate your maximum heart rate. One of the simplest is to subtract your age in years from 220, but unfortunately this method is far from accurate, due to differences in individuals and their heart size. A smaller heart beats more quickly than a larger heart size. This results in an individual with a small heart reaching their maximum heart rate too early, which will hold them back from working as hard as they could. On the other hand, an individual with a larger heart will find it difficult to reach their maximum heart rate using this calculation, resulting in them over-training in a session. The fact is that your maximum heart rate can vary, depending on what exercise or machine you are using, so a more accurate way to calculate your maximum heart rate is to do a simple fitness test on the machine of your choice – the indoor rowing machine.

To identify your maximum heart rate on a rowing machine, it is best to do the following:

- Rest for one or two days before the test.
- Do a steady warm-up on the machine for five to ten minutes at 20–24spm (strokes per minute)
- Work hard for four to eight minutes at 28–35spm with the last minute of work at your maximum effort at above 35spm.
- Record the highest your heart rate was during the test.
- This is your maximum heart rate.
- It is worthwhile repeating this test regularly, to make sure that you are still setting the correct heart rate zones for your current fitness level and getting the most out of your indoor rowing training sessions.

Calculating Heart Rate Zones

If you want to work at the right intensity on an indoor rowing machine, you need to calculate your own personal heart rate zones in order to identify the aerobic low zone, the threshold medium zone and the anaerobic high zone. Most heart rate monitors available will normally calculate this for you, but always double-check the zones with your own calculations, using the Karvonen formula. All heart rate monitors will allow you to reset the zones if and when you need to.

Karvonen Formula

(HRmax – HRrest) [×] % exercise intensity + HRrest

The Karvonen formula can be used to identify your personal heart rate zones, as shown in the following example, which gives the rate for the aerobic low zone:

195 (HRmax) – 60 (HRrest) = 135
so,
135 [×] 0.60 (60% of exercise intensity) = 81
81 + 60 (HRrest) = 141

Therefore 60% of your maximum heart rate is 141bpm.

Heart Rate Zones

Aerobic Low Zone

This zone is 60–80% of your maximum heart rate and is commonly used in three different indoor rowing workout sessions: the active recovery session, the slow and long session, and the tempo session. Active recovery sessions are at the lower end of the heart rate range and should only be used when your body is tired and you are trying to aid recovery, or when you are bringing your heart rate back down between faster-paced bursts in a higher intensity indoor rowing workout. An active recovery should be around 60% of your maximum heart rate. Slow and long sessions will be at a pace at which you can comfortably hold a conversation. This pace will improve over time as your fitness improves, but remember to not get carried away. Slow and long sessions should be around 60–75% of your maximum heart rate. Tempo sessions will be at a pace that connects the intensity gap into the next main heart rate training zone – the threshold medium zone. When you are working at the tempo session intensity, you should not be able to hold it for much longer than fifteen minutes, but you should be able to repeat it if you drop your intensity down between each session. A tempo session interval on an indoor rowing machine is usually around ten to fifteen minutes and repeated between two and four times. The tempo session should be around 75–80% of your maximum heart rate.

Threshold Medium Zone

This zone is 80–95% of your maximum heart rate. The threshold medium zone is an intensity that would include intervals, time trials and racing workouts on the indoor rowing machine. The medium zone is where your body stops relying on oxygen at an aerobic level and starts to function at an anaerobic level. At this intensity you should find it difficult to hold a conversation, being able to say only a few words before you need to get your breath back. In the threshold medium zone your workout interval time should be forty-five seconds to four minutes, but again it can be repeated if you allow enough recovery time between each interval.

Anaerobic High Zone

This zone is 95–100% of your maximum heart rate. The anaerobic high zone involves sprinting and maximum power work on the indoor rowing machine. Depending on your fitness level, this pace would involve intervals of between ten seconds and up to one minute of maximum effort, repeated for a set number of repetitions. If you are working in this high zone then the feeling you should have is that you are not be able to talk.

Recommendations and Guidelines

The weekly guidelines and recommendations for your new fitness routine can vary, depending on your reason for starting it, but remember that anything above your current schedule will have a positive benefit. The guidelines for wanting to improve your health are as follows: five to seven days per week at a moderate intensity (enough to slightly increase your heart rate) for thirty minutes total each day. If you want to improve your fitness, though, the guidelines are different: five to seven days per week at moderate to high intensity (60–90% of your maximum heart rate) for between thirty and sixty minutes total each day. It is important to be aware that thirty to sixty minutes does not necessarily have to be continuous exercise. Three ten-minute bouts of exercise throughout the day can be just as effective as a single thirty-minute session.

The Biggest Cardio Myth: 'The Fat-Burning Zone'

Amazingly enough, there is still a widespread belief among many fitness enthusiasts that if you want to burn body-fat, then you have to work your heart rate in a magical low zone of 55–65% of your maximum heart rate. Even today, there are cardio machines in health clubs that still have a fat-burning workout button. If you want to get results quickly you should ignore it. Body-fat reduction can only take place when you burn more energy than you consume. It is that simple and not exactly a complicated science. If you burn more calories than you consume, then your body will change shape. The confusion starts because, when you work at lower heart rate intensities, your body does utilize a slightly higher percentage of fat calories, compared to carbohydrate calories; because the intensity is so low, however, your total amount of calories burnt will be low, resulting in a low number of fat calories burnt. If you work your body at a higher intensity, however, the percentage of fat calories burnt might be a little lower than before, but because you are burning more total calories in the workout session the result will be more fat calories burned.

When your goal is to drop weight or to change your body shape, try not to think too much about burning fat, but rather focus on your total calorie burn. If you keep it simple and burn more calories or energy than your body takes in, then you will see those inches drop. Another reason to keep the intensity high is how it affects Excess Post-exercise Oxygen Consumption (EPOC). EPOC is like a calorie afterburner that is started by exercise. Research shows that the higher the workout intensity, the more the body will burn calories, even after the workout. So do not be afraid to up your workout intensity when you need to, since the results will be faster.

	Fat	Carbohydrate	Total calories burned	Fat calories burned
Low intensity	55%	45%	500 calories	275 fat calories
High intensity	45%	55%	700 calories	315 fat calories

How to Train Hard

When it comes to increasing your indoor rowing workout sessions in the most effective way possible, interval training is a must. Interval training is basically a set time of high intensity (threshold medium zone or anaerobic high zone), followed by a set time in a low intensity (active rest in the aerobic low zone), and repeated for a set number of repetitions, depending on your fitness level and final goal. The secret to interval training is not necessarily about how many calories you can burn during the workout, but rather how many calories your body will continue to burn after the workout. As mentioned above, interval training has fantastic effects on the body's EPOC. If done properly, it can supercharge your fitness, boost your metabolism and burn off calories more quickly than you ever thought possible. Interval training is a must in your indoor rowing machine weekly routines, no matter what your final goal may be.

7 Benefits of Strength Training

A well-balanced resistance programme in any fitness routine, including indoor rowing, is crucial. Too many people avoid resistance training because they believe it will only result in them 'bulking up' and hindering their performance on the indoor rowing machine. This could not be further from the truth. There are many excellent reasons to include some form of resistance training into your workout routine, including stronger tendons and ligaments, improved strength, improved lean muscle, an increase in bone density, a reduction in body fat, prevention of injuries, improved posture, reduction in cholesterol and reduction in blood pressure.

Resistance Training Myths

Despite all the studies and research carried out worldwide to prove the many benefits and the truth behind resistance training, you will still hear many myths throughout the fitness community. Please never believe any of the following:

Myth One
When you stop training, all your muscle will turn into fat.

Impossible. Muscle is muscle and fat is fat. They are completely different types of body tissue. If you stop training, your muscle mass and strength will decrease and your fat store may increase if you eat more calories than you burn, but you cannot turn one into the other.

Myth Two
Resistance training will reduce your flexibility.

If you train properly and perform each resistance exercise with strict form through a full range of motion, you can maintain, and in some cases even improve, your flexibility. Doing partial repetitions and following an unbalanced resistance training programme is the only way that you could possibly reduce flexibility, as well as risk injury.

Myth Three
If women include any sort of resistance training in their fitness programme, they will get big and look like a bodybuilder.

Resistance training is only a small part of changing your body shape successfully. Diet and family genetics are major factors. Regular resistance training will improve muscle tone and definition, but getting physically bigger comes down to a lot of hard training and a lot of eating. Women can never achieve the same muscle bulk as a man, due to their lower levels of testosterone, so turning into a bodybuilder is very unlikely.

Myth Four
Resistance training will damage your joints.

Regular resistance training will strengthen your ligaments and tendons, which will result in stronger, more stable joints. Rarely will a resistance programme have much, if any, impact on it, so the low-impact nature of the training will place less stress on the joint than a high-impact exercise will do.

Types of Resistance Training

Resistance training, depending on your goals, body type and exercise history, can be simplified into three main categories: endurance, strength and power. The exercise itself does not necessarily determine which category you are training in, but rather how much weight you are lifting, the speed at which you are lifting and how many times you are lifting it. To get the benefits of muscular endurance, you should be lifting a light-to-moderate weight that you can manage for a higher number of repetitions at a steady pace. Generally, when it comes to muscular strength, you will gain strength benefits if you use heavier weights that you can manage for a lower repetition range at a slower pace. For muscular power, the main factor that you should take into consideration is to do the exercise movement at a fast explosive pace. Muscular power can involve a light, moderate or heavy weight, as long as you feel in control of it for the desired repetitions.

Core Training and Posture

Core training is important in any fitness programme. Your core is your centre of gravity and every move you make starts in your core. If you decide to leave out core training in your indoor rowing fitness programme, you will miss out on all of the benefits, including improved power, agility, balance and a toned mid-section, as well as improved posture, which can help to reduce the risk of injuries to your lower back and spine. Good posture will ensure that you will be able to perform each resistance exer-

cise or movement with minimal strain on your joints, muscles and internal organs. On the other hand, bad posture can quickly result in joint or muscular injury. Continued bad posture over a long period can even lead to osteoarthritis in later life.

What Can Cause Poor Posture?

Poor posture can be caused by a number of factors. Some of the main reasons include:

• Being overweight.
• Muscular imbalances.
• Bad diet.
• Past injuries.
• Bad footwear.
• Pregnancy.
• Foot problems.

Testing Your Posture

The good news is that if you have any muscular imbalances that cause bad posture, there is a simple test you can carry out with a friend to see what areas are tight and what areas are weak. You can then transfer the results to your individual resistance programme. For example, if your hip flexors are tight and your glutes are weak, this can lead to your pelvis tilting forward (very common with people who sit down a lot in their jobs). To combat this you should concentrate on stretching your hip flexors and strengthening your glutes or buttocks.

Overhead Squat Test

The overhead squat test is one of the simpler methods to check your posture. To make sure you can see any muscular imbalances you may have, it is worthwhile getting the help of a friend to take a short video of you doing the move from three different viewpoints: front, side and back. This style of test is useful at the start of a new indoor rowing fitness programme as it will help you to not overtrain areas of your body that are already tight. As your training develops and changes, then so will your body, so it is a good idea to carry out the following overhead squat test regularly (once a month is more than enough), since muscular imbalances can change over time.

The Move
- Start in a relaxed position with your feet shoulder-width apart.
- Raise both arms above your head, keeping them next to your ears, if possible.
- Perform the squat by bending your knees and lowering yourself down as if you were sitting on a chair, then return back up to the start position.
- Throughout the move keep both arms up high.
- Repeat the move at a steady pace for ten to twenty repetitions.

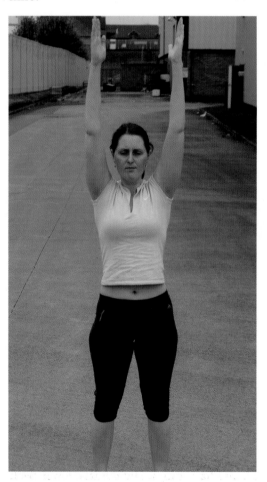

Overhead squat test: reach as high as you can at the start of the move.

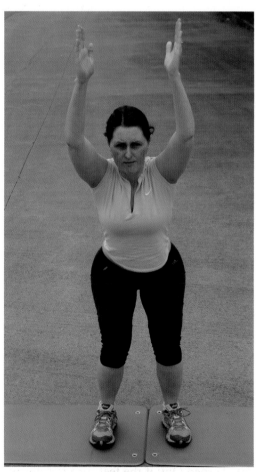

Overhead squat test: perform the squat to see which muscles are tight.

Checklist

This is where it makes sense to recruit a fitness professional to assess the movement. If that is not an option, however, you should train your eye to look out for abnormal movements throughout your own body movement. A friend with a video camera is useful, since you can use the resulting footage to check your squat over and over again. To keep the checklist as simple as possible, it has been simplified to cover five different check points of the body. It starts from ground level and works its way up the body: feet, knees, hips, shoulders and head. The perfect position throughout the overhead squat assessment is as follows: your feet stay grounded with your toes facing forward, your knees should stay in line with your big toe and second toe, your hips should remain centred without your back arching or rounding, your arms should stay high and straight, and, finally, your head should not drop forward. Unfortunately, due to our lifestyles, it is very rare to see the perfect overhead squat. It is unusual to find anyone where at least one area of the body is not more dominant, causing muscular imbalances that need to be addressed.

Every observation during the overhead squat assessment will have a problem area, and every problem area will have an exercise solution that can help to reduce the problem. Any muscle that is too tight needs to be addressed with the appropriate muscle stretch (see Chapter 5); the weak areas can be addressed with the appropriate resistance exercises, which can all be found in the same chapter. The list of abnormal movements that can be spotted during an overhead squat test is quite long. The more common muscular imbalances are listed below.

Feet

Feet Turned Out: if the feet turn out during the overhead squat assessment, then the chances are that your lower calf, hamstring and outer thigh could be tight and need to be stretched. The glutes or buttocks could be weak and need to be strengthened (the bridge exercise is an effective way to strengthen your glutes).

Heels Lifted: if the heels lift up, then it is a sign that all of the calf muscle is tight and needs to be stretched. The shin muscles could be weak and require strengthening (to strengthen the shin muscles, walk a short distance with your weight on your heels and toes lifted up off the floor).

Knees

Knees Cave In: if one, or both, knees starts to cave in during the overhead squat assessment move, then the main area that could be tight and needs to be stretched is your inner thigh. The glutes could be weak (perform the bridge exercise).

Knees Bow Out: if the knees move out of alignment during the move, then your hamstrings and outer thigh are the two main areas that could be too tight and need to be stretched. As before, the glutes could be weak (perform the bridge exercise).

Hips

Hips Shift to One Side: when the hips shift more to one side as you squat down then there can be many tight areas that need to be stretched, including calf, hamstring, inner thighs and outer thighs. The weak areas could be your glutes and deep internal abdominals (perform the bridge exercise and the plank exercise).

Lower Back Arches: when the lower back arches it is known as an anterior tilt. The areas that are too tight and need stretching are the hamstrings, abdominals, lower back and the side of the back. The weak area is your glutes (perform the bridge exercise).

Lower Back Rounds: when the lower back rounds during the overhead squat assessment, it is known as a posterior tilt. The areas that are too tight and need to be stretched are the abdominals, obliques (side of the stomach) and hamstrings. The weak area is your glutes (perform the bridge exercise).

Shoulders

Arms Fall Forward: when both arms fall forward as you squat down, the two areas that are too tight and need to be stretched are the chest and side of your back. The areas that are too weak and need to be strengthened are the middle and upper back area (perform the cobra exercise).

Elbows Bend: when your arms bend as you squat down, the tight area that needs to be stretched is the chest area. As before, the weak areas that need to be strengthened are the middle and upper back (perform the cobra exercise).

Head

Head Dips Forward: when the head falls forward as you perform the overhead squat assessment move, it is a sign that your neck muscles are too tight and need to be stretched. The weak muscle that needs to be strengthened is the deep cervical flexors (to strengthen this area all you have to do keep your chin tucked in).

Exercise Library

The following library of resistance exercises is specific to the sport of indoor rowing. More importantly, however, each section has a choice of resistance exercises that you can do, no matter which piece of fitness equipment you may have for your workout session at that time: stability ball, medicine ball, dumb-bells, resistance band or just your body weight.

Total Body Exercises

Stability Ball

Squat Thrust Press. Position yourself with your shins on top of the stability ball, making sure both hands are on the ground, shoulder-width apart. From this press-up position, with your abs drawn in tight, the move is as follows: bring both knees in towards the chest and then return them to the start position; following that, lower your upper body down to the ground by doing a press-up and return back up to the start position to repeat.

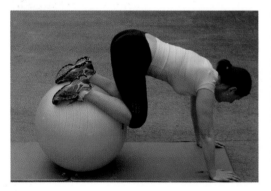

Squat thrust press: remember to tense your stomach as you bring both knees in.

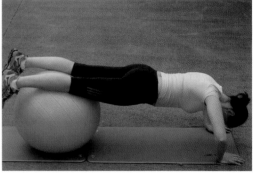

Squat thrust press: keep your back straight as you perform the press-up.

Medicine Ball

Squat with Pendulum: start with both feet a hip-width apart and, remembering to keep both arms straight, hold on to the medicine ball. As you squat down, allow the medicine ball to drop and swing in between the legs. As you drive up, allow the body momentum to swing the medicine ball up to shoulder or head height, before returning back to the start position to repeat.

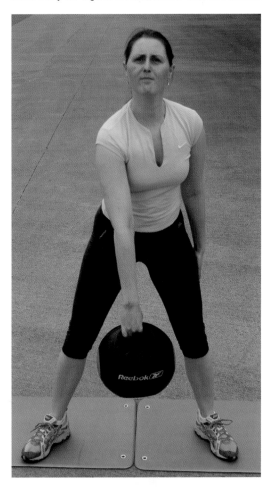

Squat with pendulum: allow the ball to swing between the legs as you lower your body.

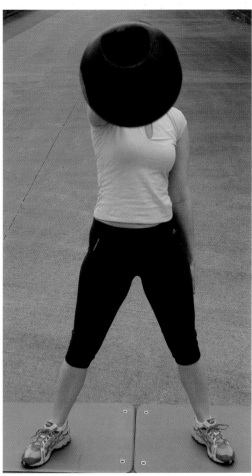

Squat with pendulum: straighten and keep the arm straight as the ball swings up.

Dumb-bells

Squat with High Pull: start again with both feet a hip-width apart with both dumb-bells held at arm's length in front of the body. From here, squat down, keeping your chest high and abs drawn in. As the body returns back to the top, pull both dumb-bells up high, remembering to keep the dumb-bells close to the body. Both elbows should not go any higher than shoulder height and the dumb-bells should go no higher than around chest level. Return the dumb-bells back to the start position and repeat.

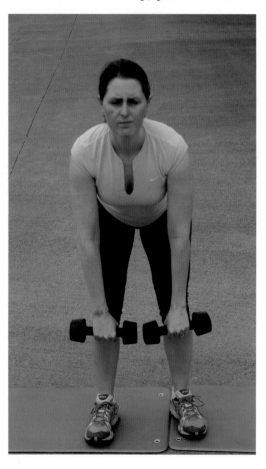

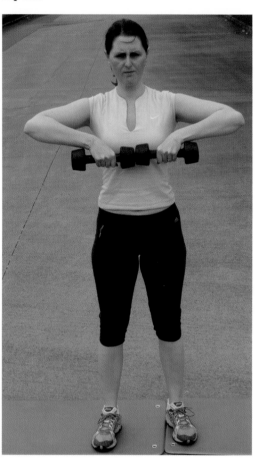

Squat with high pull: don't let the dumb-bells go much lower than your knees.

Squat with high pull: the target for the dumb-bells should be the middle of your chest.

Resistance Band

Squat with Row: first check that the resistance band is securely fastened around a door handle or post. Start with both feet a hip-width apart and, while holding on to the resistance band, walk back until there is enough tension in the band. From here, squat down, pushing your buttocks back and keeping your chest high throughout the move. As you stand back up, pull the resistance band in towards your body and slowly return to the start position and repeat.

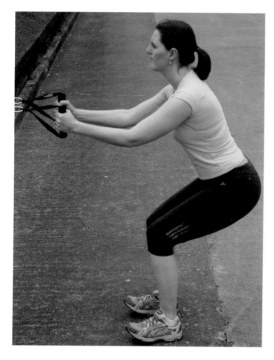

Squat with row: sit the weight back into the squat, keeping tension in the band.

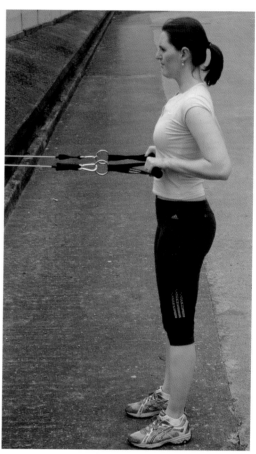

Squat with row: pull the band in as you start to stand back up.

Body weight

Burpee: start in a standing position. From here, bend both knees and bring the body down towards the ground, placing both hands out in front on the ground. Kick both legs behind into a press-up position and back in, then stand back up to the start position and repeat.

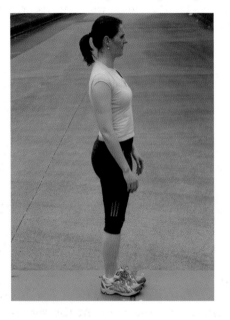

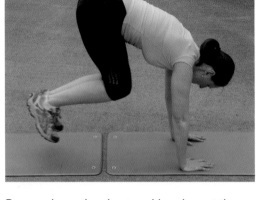

Burpee: keep the chest and head up at the start of the move.

Burpee: lower your hands and kick out and in, before returning to the top.

Core Exercises

Stability Ball

Bridge: position the body on a stability ball, so that both your shoulder blades and head are supported by the ball. The feet should be a hip-width apart on the ground and both hands should be placed on the hips. From here, slowly lower your hips down towards the ground and then push back up to the top, remembering to tense your abs and buttocks at the top of the move, before lowering again and repeating.

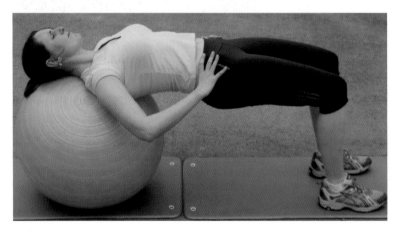

Bridge: squeeze your buttocks at the top of the move.

Medicine Ball

Seated Twist: start by sitting on the floor, with the knees bent and both feet on the ground. From here, slowly lean back with the medicine ball to an arm's length distance away from the knees. Tuck the chin in towards your chest and begin to twist the upper body to one side with the medicine ball, remembering not to allow your feet to leave the floor. Return to the centre and repeat on the other side for the desired number of repetitions.

Seated twist: look to the side where you are twisting the medicine ball.

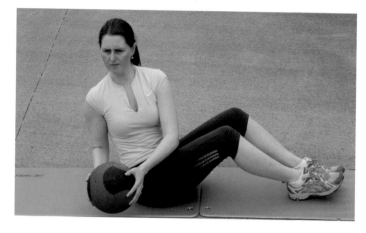

Dumb-bells

Crunch and Punch: start by laying down on your back with the knees bent and both feet on the ground, holding on to one or two dumb-bells. Pick a focal point above you and slowly lift the shoulders off the floor, remembering to keep your head steady throughout the move. Do not lift them so high that the lower back loses contact with the floor. At the top of the crunch, hold the position and slowly punch the dumb-bell out in front of you, return the dumb-bell back to your chest and then lower back down to the start position and repeat.

Crunch and punch: keep the lower back down as the shoulders lift up.

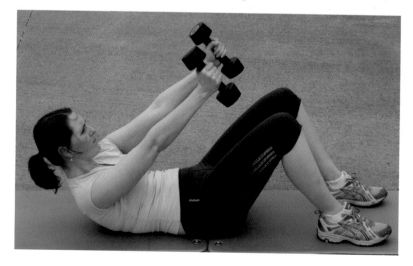

Resistance Band

Woodchop: make sure the resistance band has been fixed to a secure point. Start in a standing position, holding on to the resistance band with both hands by one side of the body. Move out to the point where there is tension in the resistance band. From here, slowly rotate the body to the other side, allowing both arms to bring the band from a low to a high position. Return to the start position and repeat.

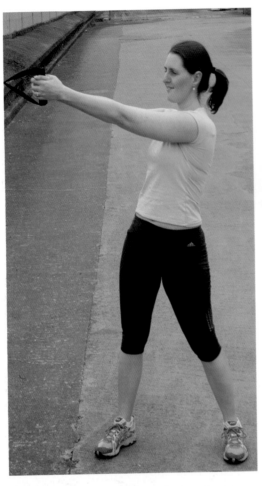

Woodchop: keep tension in the band at the top of the move.

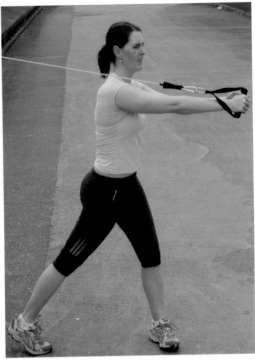

Woodchop: pivot on one foot and keep the arms straight as you rotate.

OPPOSITE: Leg curls: dig your heels into the ball as you curl it in towards you.

Body weight

The Plank: start by lying down on your stomach on the floor. Place both elbows underneath your shoulders. Resting on both forearms, slowly lift the body up into a straight line and hold this position for a few seconds, remembering to keep your abs and buttocks tight, before returning back down to the floor and repeating.

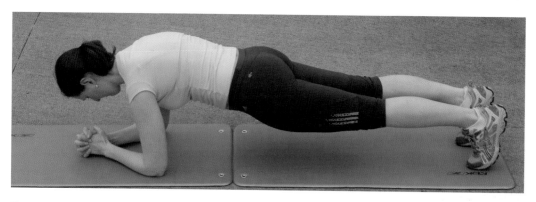

The Plank: tighten up your abs, buttocks and thighs for best results.

Leg Exercises

Stability Ball

Leg Curls: start by laying down on your back on the floor with both heels up on the stability ball. Place both hands on the floor and lift your body up into a straight line, remembering to keep abs and buttocks tight. Only if you feel in control of this position can you then start the move. Start by curling both heels in towards the buttocks, allowing the ball to move in as you curl. Keep the hips high throughout the move. Slowly extend the legs back out and repeat.

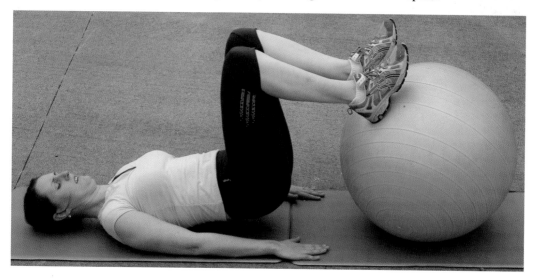

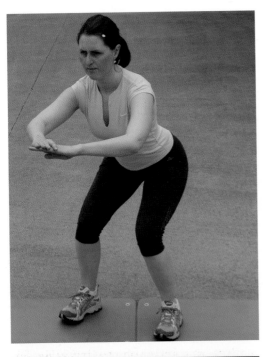

Medicine Ball

Squat: start in a standing position with both feet hip-width apart, holding on to the medicine ball at chest level. Sit back into the squat move, keeping your chest high, as if sitting on a seat. Go as low as is comfortable for you, then return back to the top and repeat.

Squat: the chest should stay up as your hips move back and down.

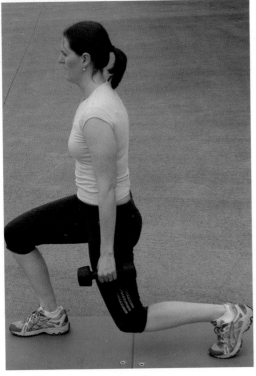

Dumb-bells

Alternating Lunges: holding on to the dumb-bells by your side and keeping your feet a hip-width apart, step one foot forward and drop the body weight down into a straight line, leading with the back knee. Keep your weight in the centre and do not allow your front knee to go over the toes. Return back up to the top and then repeat on the other leg.

Alternating lunges: lead the move with your back knee straight down to the floor.

Resistance Band

Squat: start in a standing position with both feet a hip-width apart. Both feet should be on the resistance band, while you hold both handles of the band up at shoulder level. From here, sit back into a squatting position, remembering to keep your chest high throughout the move, and then return back up to the top and repeat.

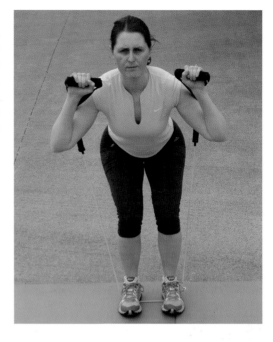

RIGHT: Squat: make sure both feet are on top of the band.

BELOW: Squat jump: start with a small squat, sitting the hips back.

BELOW RIGHT: Squat jump: explode up and jump, reaching as high as you can.

Body weight

Squat Jump: start in a standing position, with your feet a hip-width apart. Sit back into a squatting position, then drive up quickly into a straight jump into the air, reaching as high as you can during the lift. When you land back down into the start position, remember to land with bent knees, and then repeat.

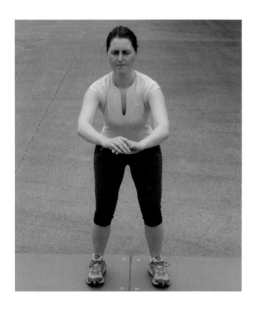

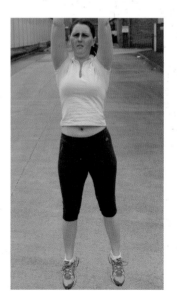

Chest Exercises

Stability Ball
Stability Press-Up: place both hands on either side of the stability ball, remembering to keep your wrists straight. Then lift your body up into a press-up position, keeping your abs tight and body line straight. Only when you feel in control of this position should you start the move. Slowly lower the chest down towards the ball by bending both arms and then return to the top to repeat.

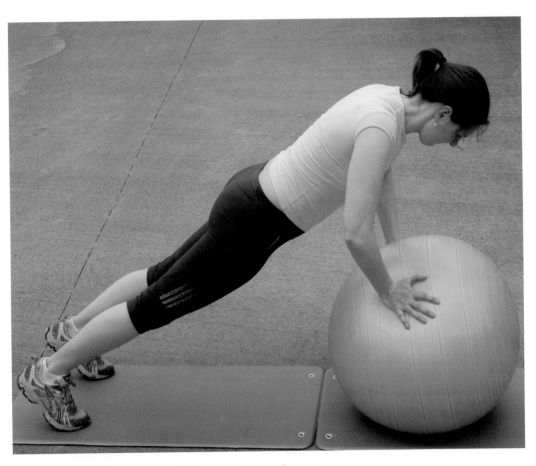

Stability press-up: keep the stomach tight as you lower yourself down to the ball.

Medicine Ball

Press-Up and Roll: start on the floor in a press-up position. With one hand on the floor, place the other hand on a medicine ball. Keeping your abs tight and body in a straight line, lower your chest down towards the floor and return to the top. Once you reach the top of the move, roll the medicine ball to the other hand and repeat the press-up.

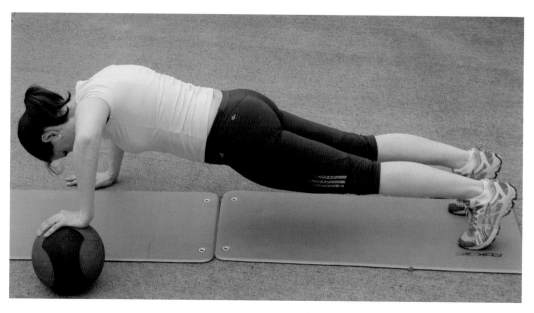

Press-up and roll: try to keep a straight line with your body as you lower yourself down.

Dumb-bells

Chest Flyes: start by laying down on the floor on your back, with a dumb-bell in each hand and both arms straight up. Keeping your abs tight, bring both arms out wide to the side, but do not rest them on the floor, before returning back up to the top to repeat. Try to keep a slight bend on both elbows throughout the move.

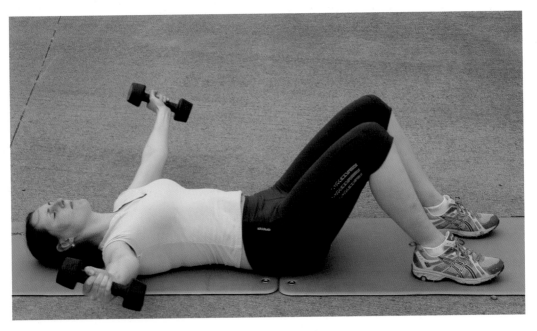

Chest flyes: remember to keep the dumb-bells level with your chest as you widen your position.

Resistance Band

Standing Chest Press: place the resistance band around your back or fasten it to a secure point. Grip both ends of the band with both hands. Stand in a split position to help support your back and slowly press both hands forward, keeping them in line with the middle of your chest, before returning back to the start position to repeat.

Body Weight

Press-Up: start on the floor with both hands outside shoulder-width. You can be on your toes, or if you prefer, you can drop to your knees for the move. Keeping your buttocks and abs tight, slowly lower the body towards the floor and press back up to the top, before repeating the move.

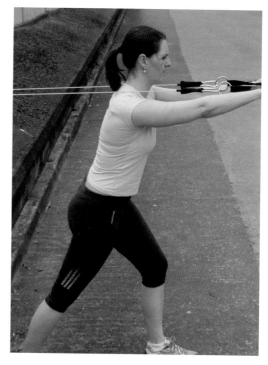

ABOVE: Standing chest press: lean your body forward slightly for better control.

BELOW: Press-up: make a triangle shape with your head and hands as you lower yourself.

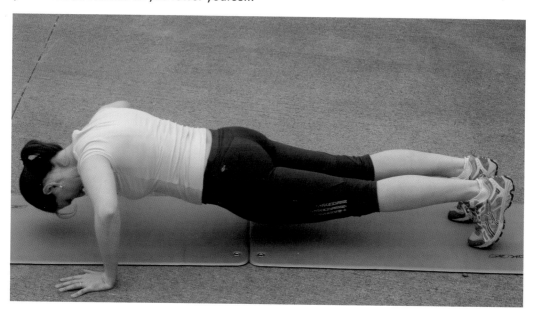

Back Exercises

Stability Ball
Cobra: position the body on top of the stability ball so that the stomach is in contact with the ball. Keep both feet in contact with the floor throughout the move and keep your chin tucked. From here, slowly lift the chest and at the same time raise both arms to the side, pinching both shoulder blades together at the top of the move. Hold the top phase for a couple of seconds before returning back down to the start position to repeat.

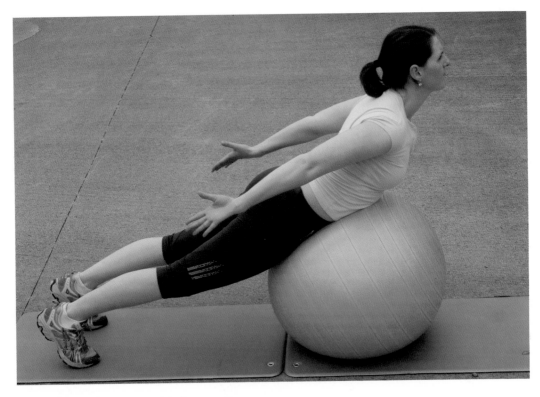

Cobra: pinch the shoulder blades together as you raise off the ball.

Medicine Ball

Bent-Over Figure Eight: start in a standing position with both feet just outside hip-width. Holding on to the medicine ball with both hands, tip from the hip and pass the ball from one hand to the other, making a figure eight between the legs. Remember to repeat the move in the other direction for balanced results.

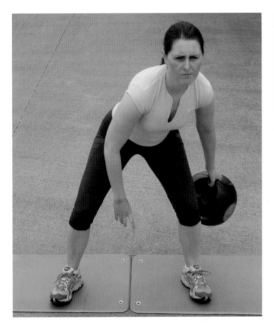

Bent-over figure eight: keep the feet grounded as the ball passes through.

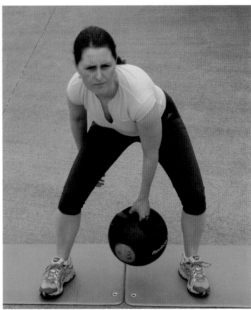

Bent-over figure eight: remain low for the best results.

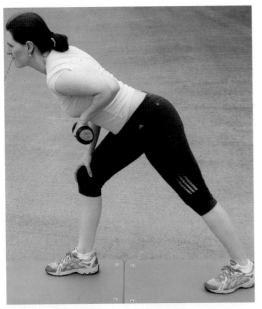

Dumb-bells

Single Arm Row: start in a standing position, with one leg further forward than the other in a split stance. Tip forward from the hip and rest one hand on the front leg. Holding on to the dumb-bell with the other hand, start to slowly pull the dumb-bell up towards the side of the upper body before returning back down to the start position to repeat.

Single arm row: keep the elbow in close to the side of your body.

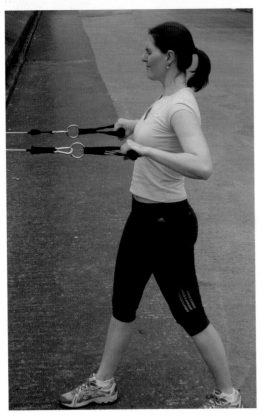

Resistance Band

Standing Row: make sure that the resistance band is fastened to a secure point. Hold on to each end of the band and walk back until you feel enough tension in the band. From this position, pull both ends of the band in towards each side of the upper body. Return back to the start position and repeat.

Standing row: squeeze the shoulder blades together as you pull the band.

Body weight

Back Raise: start by lying down on your stomach on the floor. With your hands placed by the side of your head, or on your buttocks if you prefer, slowly lift the chest up from the floor as high as is comfortable for you, remembering to keep your eyes focused on the ground. Return back down to the start position and repeat.

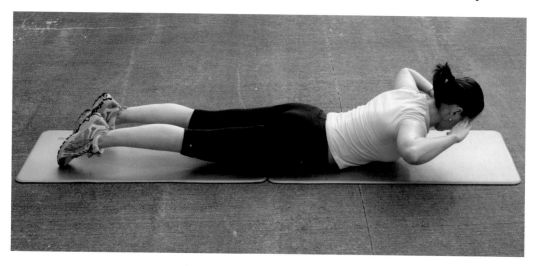

Back raise: eyes should be fixed on the floor throughout the move.

Shoulder Exercises

Stability Ball

Decline Press-Up: position yourself so that your shins, or thighs if you want it easier, are on the top of the stability ball, with both hands placed outside shoulder-width on the floor. Slowly lower the upper body down towards the floor and return back up to the top and repeat.

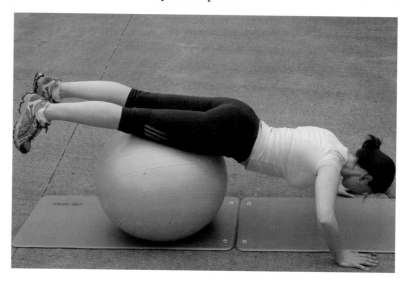

Decline press-up: for more intensity, rest your shins on the ball.

Medicine Ball
Medicine Ball Press: start in a standing position with one leg slightly further forward
than the other in a split stance. Holding on
to the medicine ball at chest height, slowly
press the ball up high, return back down to
chest level and repeat.

Dumb-bells
Upright Row: start in a standing position
with one leg slightly further forward than the
other in a split stance. Holding the dumb-
bells down in front of both thighs, slowly lift
the dumb-bells up, leading the move with
both elbows, to the middle of the chest.
Remember not to let the elbows go any
higher than your shoulders. Lower the
dumb-bells back down to the start position
and repeat.

Resistance Band
Standing Press: start in a standing position,
making sure that one, or both, feet are
securely on top of the resistance band.
Holding on to each end of the band, bring it
up to your shoulder height. From here,
slowly press both hands up above your head
and return back down to shoulder height to
repeat.

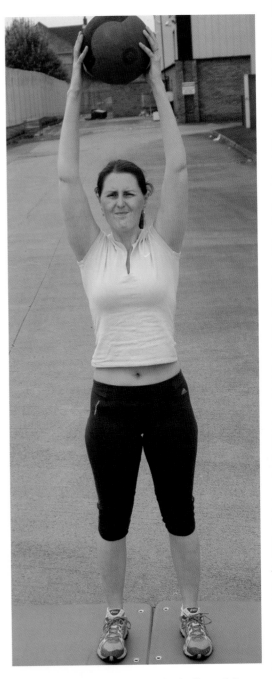

Medicine ball press: press the ball straight
up from your chin.

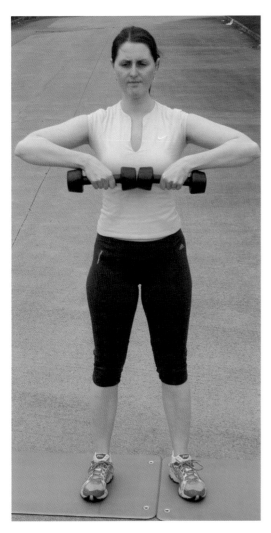

Upright row: make sure the elbows don't go any higher than your shoulders.

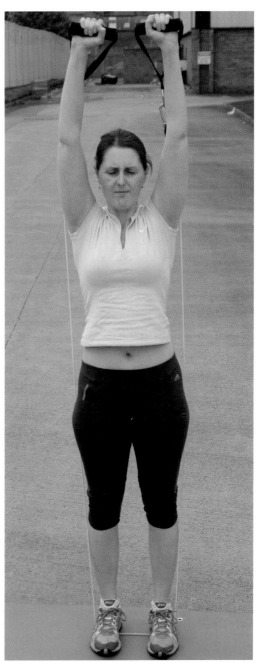

Standing press: remember to have your weight fully on the band.

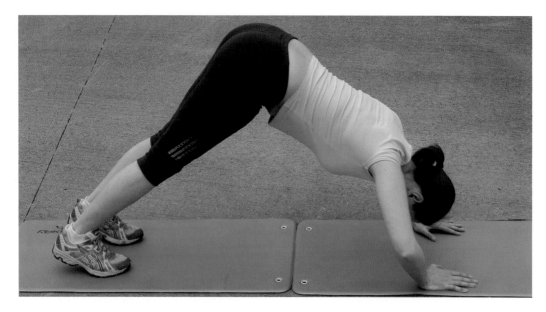

Triangle press-up: keep the hips high as you lower your
head towards the floor.

Body weight
Triangle Press-Up: start by laying down on
the floor on your stomach. With your hands
outside shoulder-width, lift your body
weight up and push your buttocks up into
the air so that the body is in a triangle position. From this triangle position, slowly bend
both arms, bringing the upper body down
towards the floor, before returning back up
to the start to repeat.

Arm Exercises

Stability Ball
Stability Dips: start by sitting on the stability
ball, with both hands on the front of the ball
for support and both feet hip-width apart on
the ground. From here, shift the body weight
forward off the stability ball, until you are
supporting your body weight with your
arms. Only when you feel in control of this
position do you start the move. Bend both
elbows back and then lower the body down
to what is comfortable for you, before
returning to the top to repeat.

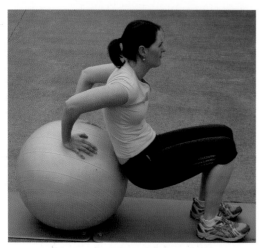

Stability dips: make sure your buttocks are in
close to the ball.

Medicine Ball

Ball Curl: start in a split stance and hold on to the medicine ball with both hands at thigh level. Slowly curl the medicine ball up towards the shoulders and return back down to the thighs to repeat.

RIGHT: Ball curl: squeeze your arms as you curl the ball from thighs to shoulders.

BELOW: Overhead ball extension: keep both elbows in tight as the ball comes back.

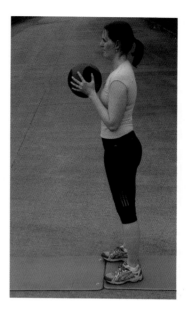

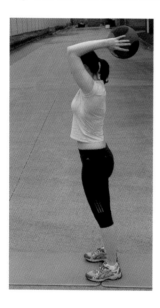

Overhead Ball Extension: start in a split stance and hold on to the medicine ball with both hands above your head. Keeping both shoulders steady, slowly bend both elbows, bringing the medicine ball back and down until the elbows are approximately at a right angle. Return back to the top and repeat.

Dumb-bells

Standing Curls: start in a standing position with both feet hip-width apart. Holding on to both dumb-bells by your side, slowly curl both dumb-bells up towards the shoulders before returning back down to repeat. Remember not to swing the body through the move.

Standing curls: check that both elbows remain close to your sides when curling.

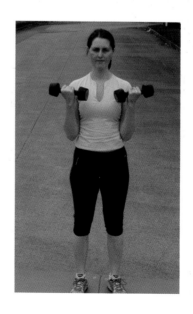

Kneeling Kickbacks: position yourself on both hands and knees on the floor, keeping the back straight and stomach tight. Hold on to one dumb-bell and bring that elbow to your side. Starting from this right angle, slowly extend back until the dumb-bell is level with the body, before returning back down to repeat. Remember not to swing from your shoulder.

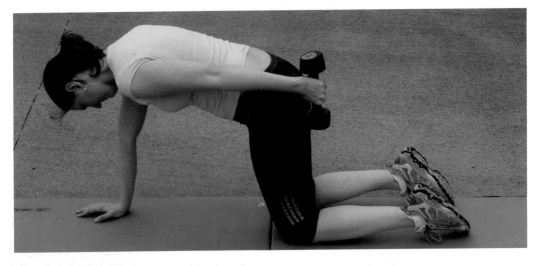

Kneeling kickbacks: try to extend back up into a straight line with your body.

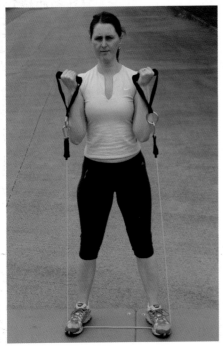

Resistance Band

Standing Curls: start in a standing position and make sure that you securely place the resistance band under both feet. Holding on to both ends of the band, bring them up by the side of your thighs. If you do not feel any tension, position both feet wider on the resistance band. From here, slowly curl both hands up towards the shoulders and return back to the side of your thighs to repeat.

Standing curls: control the band back down slowly for good results.

Single Arm Overhead Extension: start in a standing position and place one end of the resistance band under one foot and hold on to the other end with your hand. Bring the band up above the head until the arm is straight. If you need more tension in the band, place the foot further along the band to shorten its length. From here, slowly bend the elbow, bringing the band back until your elbow is at a right angle and then return to the top and repeat.

Body weight
Narrow Press-Up: start by laying on the floor on your stomach. Lift the body weight up into a straight line, keeping your hands no wider than shoulder-width apart. If you want to drop the intensity, drop to the knees for the move. From here, bend both elbows back, keeping them close to your body, lowering the upper body down towards the floor and then return back to the top and repeat.

RIGHT: Single arm overhead extension: for more intensity, shorten the band by standing further up.

BELOW: Narrow press-up: keep both elbows in tight as you lower your body down.

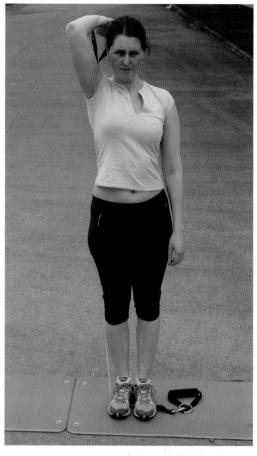

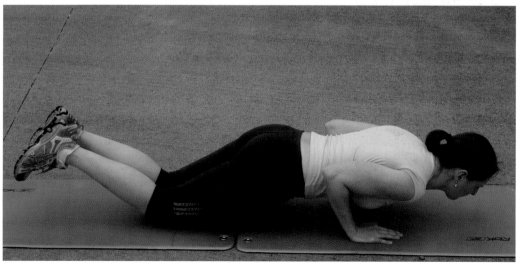

8 Indoor Rowing for Weight Loss

Weight loss has always been one of the major reasons why people first decide to change their lifestyle and start a new fitness routine. If losing weight is the reason you became involved with indoor rowing, then the chances are that you are also interested in improving your fitness level and health, as well as your physical appearance. If you believe you fall into one of these categories, this weight-loss section will help answer all your questions on how to achieve your weight-loss goal – no matter how small or big it may be. One of the main reasons why indoor rowing is an excellent way to lose weight is that its low-impact nature keeps it as one of the safest forms of exercise and, since it covers every major muscle group in the body, it is fantastic for weight loss, especially for those just starting out.

Basic Science

Fat loss is not a complicated science, even though many individuals will try to make it more complex than it actually is. The basic of losing weight and burning body fat is to burn more calories than you consume. If you take in more calories than you burn during your daily life, then you will put on weight. Keep it simple. Too many people try to complicate things by going on fad diets, many of which are usually just a short-term fix that will have you craving food down the line, with the result that you will soon be at square one

again. In short, fad diets will never work in the long run. The important thing to remember is to eat a healthy balanced diet and try not to consume more than you actually need.

One of the main reasons why people do not lose weight or reach their weight-loss goal is that they lack motivation. When many individuals first start out, they do not understand exactly what it is they should be doing to keep on the proper path. Since this is such a crucial factor when it comes to achieving the intended weight loss through indoor rowing, it is necessary to understand your motives for doing this and how it can work for you, before moving on to the weight-loss workout routines. You first need to create a plan, laying things out or writing them down in a way that works for you, to help you understand where you have come from and what you need to do on a daily and weekly basis in order to reach your goal. Reviewing what you are doing is vital if you want to see constant and consistent improvements towards your weight-loss goal. Do not think everything will be perfect, though, and that your weight-loss experience will be quick and smooth, and without any problems. When you start to review your indoor workout sessions, it is important to learn from any mistakes you make on the way, such as training at a time of day that does not work for you. Try to be honest with yourself as you plan your future indoor rowing

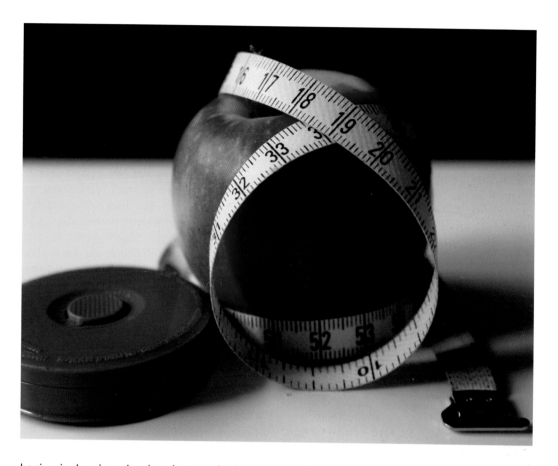

Losing inches is a simple science – don't over-complicate things.

workouts, and make sure that everything stays on track.

If you want to adopt a more active and healthier lifestyle, you need to think carefully about what you need to change about your own behaviour. When a tough situation arises and you are tempted by something, or you are just not sure what to do, imagine yourself in the shoes of the fittest person you know and decide what they would do. You might be surprised how often this keeps you on the right road to successful weight loss. As discussed above (see Chapter 4), setting down specific weight-loss targets is a critical part of achieving your new lifestyle and maintaining your indoor rowing workouts. But just writing them down is not enough. It is up to you to put every one of those goals into action. Every day you should think about how you can keep on moving forward towards your eventual goals. The trick is to break down each long-term goal into more manageable chunks. If you want to lose a lot of weight in six months, for example, think of small things that will contribute towards this on a weekly or daily basis, such as reaching a certain time or distance in your weekly indoor rowing sessions, making a point of buying certain healthy foods as part of your weekly shopping, or keeping to daily nutritional goals, which might be as simple as drinking more water. When writing down the smaller goals, you should think about your weak points and then address them. The chances are that this is not the first time you have tried to lose weight, so think about everything you might have tried before, but without success. If something did not work for you in the past, is it really going to work the second or third time round? Think of a different option or angle that you can try this time.

How Much is Too Much?

By now you should have decided on your goals, as well as the date you want to reach them by. When it comes to starting out with a new fitness plan on the indoor rowing machine, one of the big mistakes that most people make is to try to do too much too soon. Even though there are seven days to choose from every week, it is wise to start out with only two to four sessions a week, slowly building up the intensity to the point where you can exercise for the current recommended exercise guidelines for health of thirty minutes a day for five times a week. Many people are frightened at the thought of doing all thirty minutes on just an indoor rowing machine, but the good news is that it does not have to monopolize your time every day. When you are starting out, an indoor rowing machine can be just part of your thirty minutes to a new fitter lifestyle. As you become more experienced you can increase your times and intensities. For beginners, it is a good idea to use the indoor rowing machine every other day, if possible, since this will allow you to recover and get some rest between each session. You should always aim to give

yourself at least one or two days of full recovery from training when you first start out, in order to stop you overtraining and feeling stiff and sore all the time.

Body Shapes

When it comes to weight loss, a realistic time frame in which you should start to see results is eight to twelve weeks. The indoor rowing programme for weight loss will be based on this principle and will be structured over an eight-week period. To make sure you get the best results possible, and make the most of your time on the equipment, the eight-week indoor rowing programme will include suitable resistance training exercises based on your body shape.

Men's Body Shapes

Male body shapes fall into three categories: slim, heavy and athletic. If you have a naturally slim body shape, then you will have a high metabolic rate. You will have a naturally low body fat percentage and will find it difficult to increase muscle mass. On the positive side, though, dropping body fat will be very easy for you. The light body frame usually makes those with a slim body shape better suited to endurance exercises and aerobic activities.

If you have a heavy body shape, then you will have a naturally higher percentage of body fat. Your natural body frame will be larger, with most of the body fat carried around the midsection. You will have a slow metabolic rate, which will make it more difficult for you to drop body fat. If you have a heavy body shape, you can gain weight quickly and get out of condition rapidly if you decide to stop exercising for some time. Your size and weight is normally best suited for more strength-based sports and you will usually be at a disadvantage with longer endurance-based sports or exercises.

Rate of Perceived Exertion (RPE)

In terms of intensity, one of the best ways to gauge the level at which you should be working is by using the RPE scale (Rate of Perceived Exertion), which is commonly employed throughout the health and fitness industry. The scale normally goes from one to ten, and for each level on the scale there is an approximate heart rate percentage you should be working at if you like to use a heart rate monitor during your workouts. If, however, you would rather go without, there is a simpler way you can gauge the intensity you are working at – just keep an eye on how you are feeling and be aware of your breathing and your ability to talk.

RPE level 0. You are at complete rest. At this intensity you should be laying down, completely relaxed.

RPE level 1. This indicates a very light activity. You should be at this intensity when sitting down.

RPE level 2. At this intensity you are now reaching the zone where your heart rate is between 55% and 60% of your maximum heart rate. This pace should have a feeling similar to a gentle walk. You should be able to hold a comfortable conversation.

RPE level 3. At this intensity you are now reaching the zone where your heart rate is reaching 60–65% of your maximum heart rate. This pace should have a feeling that would come with a brisk walk. You would still be able to hold a comfortable conversation.

RPE level 4. At this intensity you are reaching the zone where your heart rate is reaching 65–70% of your maximum heart rate. This pace should have a feeling of a fast-paced walk, but you are still able to hold a conversation.

RPE level 5. At this intensity you are reaching the zone where your heart rate is reaching 70–75% of your maximum heart rate. This pace should again give you a feeling of a fast-paced walk, but the difference now is that you are starting to breathe a little harder.

RPE level 6. At this intensity you are approximately in the zone where your heart rate is reaching 75–80% of your maximum heart rate. This pace should give you the feeling of a light jog. You should just about be able to say a sentence or so before you have to get your breath back.

RPE level 7. At this intensity you are moving into the higher end of the scale, into the zone where your heart rate is reaching 80–85% of your maximum heart rate. This pace should give you the feeling of a faster jog or run. You should not be able to talk comfortably, having the feeling that you can hardly say one full sentence.

RPE level 8. At this intensity you are now into the zone where your heart rate is reaching 85–90% of your maximum heart rate. At this point you should feel the need to breathe more than once for each stroke. You should just about be able to say one or two words at a time, before you feel you have to get your breath back. At this level you are uncomfortable.

RPE level 9. At this intensity you are in a zone where your heart rate is at 90–95% of your maximum heart rate. You should not be able to talk. At this level you are very uncomfortable.

RPE level 10. At this intensity you are now reaching the zone where your heart rate is 95–100% of your maximum heart rate. You should not be able to hold this intensity for long and you are not able to talk at all. This is your maximum effort on the rower.

If you have an athletic body shape, then you will have wide shoulders and a narrow waist, giving your body a V-shaped appearance. Your body shape will normally be well defined and you will have a fast metabolic rate. This body shape will respond to training faster than the other two male body shapes. Those with an athletic body shape will find it easier both to increase muscle mass and to burn body fat. Due to your naturally strong, muscular look, you can sometimes fall into the trap of overtraining your muscles, leading to fatigue, so exercise at a high intensity should be moderate.

Women's Body Shapes

Female body shapes fall into four different categories: slim, curves, bottom-heavy and mid-heavy. If you fall into the slim category, your body will usually have longer limbs and your chest, waist and hips will be narrow in size. You will be lean, but your waist will be undefined. The upper body will lack any curves and you will have a relatively small waist and back. If you are a slim shape then your arms will be long and slim with noticeable definition, giving your body the illusion of being taller. Your lower body will again be lean and long with a low body fat percentage, and if you are able to tone your legs it will give you an even longer and more defined look. With a slim body shape it is unlikely you will ever be curvaceous, but you have the advantage of being one of the easiest body shapes to work with. The workout goal for the slim-shaped woman is to develop strong, well-defined shoulders – working on the upper body will give the body the illusion of curves. During a workout you should also concentrate on the waist line, making sure the midsection is strong and flat. The rear should be worked to give it more shape, again giving the illusion of more curves.

If you fall into the curves shape category, then you will have a small, curved waist and your shoulders, chest and hips will all have a similar size. Your figure will have the classic female curves. The key to keeping your body shape looking its best is to keep the waist area slim and defined. Due to the shoulders and chest already being wider than the rest of your body, they will rarely need the same exercise attention as other areas of the body. It will be beneficial for you to work your back, especially your upper back area, since this will pull back the chest, making your body shape appear taller overall. Your arms will normally require work and definition. You should also work on the hips and legs to give more shape, since the lower body area is usually where most women of this body shape feel that their curves are out of control. The workout goal for the curves-shaped woman is to slightly reduce the shape of the curves, trying to create more of a balance throughout your body. The back muscles should be worked to improve overall posture and the back of the thighs should be worked to balance out the legs and give more of a shape to the rear. Stomach work to strengthen and flatten the midsection will also help with the final balanced look.

If you fall into the bottom-heavy shape category, then you will have hips that are wider than the chest and shoulders. Even though the midsection is usually well defined, the shoulders will usually be narrow with a slim upper back, but this narrow look up top can actually lead to the lower body looking larger than it actually is. The arms tend to be long and elegant, lacking definition and shape. The hips and thighs usually store more body fat than the rest of the body, causing the bottom-heavy look, but even though this area carries more weight, it is important not to overwork this area. The workout goal for a woman in this category is to develop well-defined shoulders, which will help to slightly widen the upper body and so give the body more balance. Body fat should be reduced around the hips, rear and thighs, but this does not mean that you should constantly work the lower body. Working one area of the body too much can lead to an unbalanced look to the body.

If you have a mid-heavy shape then you will have broad shoulders, usually with smaller hips and a flat rear. The general appearance of this shape is top-heavy. You will tend to carry more weight around your midsection, compared to the other body shapes. The upper body shape of the mid-heavy woman usually has the image of being rounder and larger than the lower body, so to balance the upper and lower body it is important to concentrate on the midsection, hips and thighs during training. A woman in this category will have well-shaped arms, but the upper arms may appear to be carrying more body fat, especially around the chest area. Even though this is the main area where you will first put on weight, it is also one of the easiest places from which to lose it. The broad shoulders and back will also tend to carry quite a bit of body fat, adding to the heavy body shape look. The workout goal for the mid-heavy shaped woman is reduce body fat in the upper body area, while toning and shaping the lower body to give a more balanced appearance. It is important to emphasize the good points – the legs and the rear.

Eight-Week Weight Loss Programmes

The eight-week indoor rowing programme for weight loss is divided into three main areas: indoor rowing sessions, resistance sessions (these differ depending on your body type) and flexibility sessions. Before following the eight-week programme, please make sure you know your body shape and which resistance exercises are required (details of all the resistance exercises may be found in Chapter 7). Each body shape is assigned two different resistance workouts that you need to perform in a single week. Resistance routine one in each case will be based on the theory of horizontal loading and comprises basic repetitions and sets: you perform the given repetitions for the exercise, rest for the given time, and then perform the same exercise again, repeating it for your given number of sets. When you have finished all the sets for that exercise, you then move on to the next.

Resistance routine two in each case will be based on the principles of vertical loading, which is very similar to circuit training: you perform the given number of repetitions for that exercise and then, after minimum rest, you move straight on to the next exercise in sequence. Work your way down all of the exercises listed. Once you reach the last exercise on the list, you rest for the given time and then start back to the top of the list, before repeating back down the exercise list for the given number of vertical load sets.

The exercises require the following equipment: dumb-bells (DB), medicine ball (MB), resistance band (Band) and stability ball (Ball).

Men – Slim Shape

Resistance Routine 1
You should aim for a range of 8–12 repetitions on each exercise for 2–3 sets on each; rest for 60–90 seconds between each exercise.
(DB) Squat and High Pull
(Ball) Squat Thrust and Press
(DB) Alternating Lunges
(DB) Chest Flyes
(DB) One Arm Row
(MB) Seated Twist

Resistance Routine 2

You should aim for a range of 12–20 repetitions on each exercise, rest for 10–20 seconds and move on to the next exercise, repeating down the list. When finished, rest for 30–60 seconds and repeat all again from two to five times.

Burpees
Squat Jumps
The Plank
Press-ups
Back Raise

Men – Heavy Shape

Resistance Routine 1

You should aim for a range of 20–25 repetitions on each exercise for 2–3 sets on each. Rest for 30–60 seconds between each exercise.

(DB) Alternating Lunges
(DB) Chest Flyes
(MB) Squat
(DB) One Arm Row
(Ball) Leg Curl
The Plank

Resistance Routine 2

You should aim for a range of 12–20 repetitions on each exercise, rest for 10–20 seconds and move on to the next exercise, repeating down the list. When finished, rest for 30–60 seconds and repeat all again between two and five times.

(MB) Squat Pendulum
(MB) Squat to High Pull
(Band) Squat and Row
Burpee
(Band) Woodchop

Men – Athletic Shape

Resistance Routine 1

You should aim for a range of 10–15 repetitions on each exercise for 2–3 sets on each.

Rest for 60–90 seconds between each exercise.

Squat Jump
Press-up
(DB) One Arm Row
(DB) Upright Row
(MB) Seated Twist

Resistance Routine 2

You should aim for a range of 12–20 repetitions on each exercise, rest for 10–20 seconds and move on to the next exercise, repeating down the list. When finished, rest for 30–60 seconds and repeat all again between two and five times.

(MB) Squat Pendulum
(MB) Seated Twist
(MB) Squat
(MB) Press-up and Roll
(MB) Figure 8
(MB) Press-up

Women – Slim Shape

Resistance Routine 1

You should aim for a range of 8–12 repetitions on each exercise for 2–3 sets on each. Rest for 60–90 seconds between each exercise.

(Ball) Bridge
(DB) Punch and Crunch
(Ball) Leg Curl
(DB) Chest Flyes
(Ball) Cobra
(DB) Upright Row

Resistance Routine 2

You should aim for a range of 12–20 repetitions on each exercise, rest for 10–20 seconds and move on to the next exercise, repeating down the list. When finished, rest for 30–60 seconds and repeat all again between two and five times.

(DB) Squat and High Pull
(MB) Squat Pendulum

(Ball) Squat Thrust and Press
Burpee
The Plank

Women – Curves Shape

Resistance Routine 1
You should aim for a range of 12–20 repetitions on each exercise for 2–3 sets on each. Rest for 30–60 seconds between each exercise.
Press-up
(Ball) Leg Curl
Back Raise
(Band) Woodchop
The Plank

Resistance Routine 2
You should aim for a range of 12–20 repetitions on each exercise, rest for 10–20 seconds and move on to the next exercise, repeating down the list. When finished, rest for 30–60 seconds and repeat all again between two and five times.
(Ball) Cobra
(DB) Chest Flyes
Burpee
(Ball) Bridge

Women – Bottom-Heavy Shape

Resistance Routine 1
You should aim for a range of 20–25 repetitions on each exercise for 2–3 sets on each. Rest for 30–60 seconds between each exercise.
Burpee
(MB) Squat Pendulum
(DB) Squat and High Pull
(Ball) Bridge
The Plank
(DB) Punch and Crunch
(Ball) Cobra

Resistance Routine 2
You should aim for a range of 12–20 repetitions on each exercise, rest for 10–20 seconds and move on to the next exercise, repeating down the list. When finished, rest for 30–60 seconds and repeat all again between two and five times.
Burpee
(DB) Squat High Pull
(MB) Squat Pendulum
(Band) Woodchop
(DB) Punch and Crunch

Women – Mid-Heavy Shape

Resistance Routine 1
You should aim for a range of 20–25 repetitions on each exercise for 2–3 sets on each. Rest for 30–60 seconds between each exercise.
(MB) Squat Pendulum
(DB) Squat and High Pull
Burpees
(Ball) Squat Thrust and Press
(Ball) Bridge
The Plank

Resistance Routine 2
You should aim for a range of 12–20 repetitions on each exercise, rest for 10–20 seconds and move on to the next exercise, repeating down the list. When finished, rest for 30–60 seconds and repeat all again between two and five times.
(DB) Alternating Lunges
Press-up
(Ball) Leg Curl
(Ball) Cobra
Squat Jump
(MB) Press
(DB) Punch and Crunch

Rowing Sessions
The following list of indoor rowing machine sessions is a basic layout, based

on a maximum of four weekly workouts, that should kick-start your weight-loss mission:

• One steady-paced medium row.
• One slow-paced long row.
• One session of fast-paced short row intervals.
• One session of fast-paced long row intervals.

In addition, the eight-week indoor rowing weight loss plan includes two resistance workouts, selected according to your body shape (see above). As the weeks progress with the plan, you should be challenging yourself with your resistance workouts by attempting to increase the amount of weight you are lifting. Each indoor rowing session has a pace that is measured in strokes per minute (spm). Every indoor rowing machine should be able to show your spm on its computer display. To give yourself the best possible chance of results, make sure that your eating habits are healthy (see Chapter 13). Remember to warm up, cool down and stretch for every workout session in the eight-week plan.

Advice for Beginners

If you do not have any sort of exercise back-ground and your fitness history is not the best, then you will be starting from the beginning. Before committing yourself to an exercise routine on an indoor rowing machine, see a health professional and get a basic health check. When first starting out the prospect of the eight-week weight loss plan can be very daunting, but don't panic, because you can pick and mix some of the workouts to suit your lifestyle and current fitness level. Some individuals, for example, might find it difficult to row constantly for twenty minutes, but you can probably manage five minutes in one go and then repeat this three more times. As long as your total time equals what is asked of you, there is no problem breaking up the longer times into more manageable chunks. Another important point to remember when starting out is that every little bit helps: if you cannot manage four to five days each week, then cut back and do two to three days. Remember that the key to getting good results is to create consistency with your workouts. It is better to do three days every week than do six sessions on the first week, nothing the next week and maybe only one session the following week. Make your indoor rowing routine a habit.

Eight-Week Weight Loss Plan

Week One

Day One (Steady-Paced Medium Row)
• 10 minutes at 24–26spm. Your RPE for the session should be 7–8 out of 10.

Day Two (Fast-Paced Long Intervals)
• 3 minutes hard at 28–30spm / 3 minutes rest. Repeat three times. Your RPE for the hard section should be 8–9 out of 10.
• Resistance routine 1.

Day Three
• Complete rest

Day Four (Slow-Paced Long Row)
• 10 minutes at 18–22spm Your RPE for this session should be 6–7 out of 10.

Day Five (Short-Paced Short Intervals)
• 1 minute hard at 30–32spm / 2 minutes easy at 18–22spm. Repeat three times. Your RPE for the hard section should be 8–9 out of 10.

Day Six (Active Rest)
- Spend 20–45 minutes doing any other activity or sport, apart from indoor rowing.
- Resistance routine 2.

Day Seven
- Complete rest.

Week Two
Day One (Steady-Paced Medium Row)
- 10 minutes at 24–26spm. Your RPE for the session should be 7–8 out of 10.

Day Two (Fast-Paced Long Intervals)
- 3 minutes hard at 28–30spm / 3 minutes rest. Repeat four times. Your RPE for the hard section should be 8–9 out of 10.
- Resistance routine 1.

Day Three
- Complete rest

Day Four (Slow-Paced Long Row)
- 15 minutes at 18–22spm. Your RPE for this session should be 6–7 out of 10.

Day Five (Short-Paced Short Intervals)
- 1 minute hard at 30–32spm / 2 minutes easy at 18–22spm. Repeat four times. Your RPE for the hard section should be 8–9 out of 10.

Day Six (Active Rest)
- Spend 20–45 minutes doing any other activity or sport, apart from indoor rowing.
- Resistance routine 2.

Day Seven
- Complete rest.

Week Three
Day One (Steady-Paced Medium Row)
- 15 minutes at 24–26spm. Your RPE for the session should be 7–8 out of 10.

Day Two (Fast-Paced Long Intervals)
- 3 minutes hard at 28–30spm / 3 minutes rest. Repeat five times. Your RPE for the hard section should be 8–9 out of 10.
- Resistance routine 1 (if possible, increase your weights).

Day Three
- Complete rest.

Day Four (Slow-Paced Long Row)
- 20 minutes at 18–22spm. Your RPE for this session should be 6–7 out of 10.

Day Five (Short-Paced Short Intervals)
- 1 minute hard at 30–32spm / 2 minutes easy at 18–22spm. Repeat five times. Your RPE for the hard section should be 8–9 out of 10.

Day Six (Active Rest)
- Spend 30–45 minutes doing any other activity or sport, apart from indoor rowing.
- Resistance routine 2 (if possible, increase your weights).

Day Seven
- Complete rest.

Week Four
Day One (Steady-Paced Medium Row)
- 15 minutes at 24–26spm. Your RPE for the session should be 7–8 out of 10.

Day Two (Fast-Paced Long Intervals)
- 3 minutes hard at 28–30spm / 3 minutes rest. Repeat six times. Your RPE for the hard section should be 8–9 out of 10.
- Resistance routine 1.

Day Three
- Complete rest

Day Four (Slow-Paced Long Row)
- 25 minutes at 18–22spm. Your RPE for this session should be 6–7 out of 10.

Day Five (Short-Paced Short Intervals)
• 1 minute hard at 30–32spm / 2 minutes easy at 18–22spm) Repeat six times. Your RPE for the hard section should be 8–9 out of 10.

Day Six (Active Rest)
• Spend 30–45 minutes doing any other activity or sport, apart from indoor rowing.
• Resistance routine 2.

Day Seven
• Complete rest.

Week Five

Day One (Steady-Paced Medium Row)
• 20 minutes at 24–26spm Your RPE for the session should be 7–8 out of 10.

Day Two (Fast-Paced Long Intervals)
• 4 minutes hard at 28–30spm / 4 minutes rest. Repeat three times. Your RPE for the hard section should be 8–9 out of 10.
• Resistance routine 1 (if possible, increase your weights).

Day Three
• Complete rest.

Day Four (Slow-Paced Long Row)
• 30 minutes at 18–22spm. Your RPE for this session should be 6–7 out of 10.

Day Five (Short-Paced Short Intervals)
• 1 minute hard at 30–32spm / 1 minute easy at 18–22spm) Repeat six times. Your RPE for the hard section should be 8–9 out of 10.

Day Six (Active Rest)
• Spend 30–60 minutes doing any other activity or sport, apart from indoor rowing.
• Resistance routine 2 (if possible, increase your weights).

Day Seven
• Complete rest.

Week Six

Day One (Steady-Paced Medium Row)
• 20 minutes at 24–26spm. Your RPE for the session should be 7–8 out of 10.

Day Two (Fast-Paced Long Intervals)
• 4 minutes hard at 28–30spm / 4 minutes rest. Repeat four times. Your RPE for the hard section should be 8–9 out of 10.
• Resistance routine 1.

Day Three
• Complete rest.

Day Four (Slow-Paced Long Row)
• 35 minutes at 18–22spm Your RPE for this session should be 6–7 out of 10.

Day Five (Short-Paced Short Intervals)
• 1 minute hard at 30–32spm / 1 minute easy at 18–22spm. Repeat six times. Your RPE for the hard section should be 8–9 out of 10.

Day Six (Active Rest)
• Spend 30–60 minutes doing any other activity or sport, apart from indoor rowing.
• Resistance routine 2.

Day Seven
• Complete rest.

Week Seven

Day One (Steady-Paced Medium Row)
• 25 minutes at 24–26 spm. Your RPE for the session should be 7–8 out of 10.

Day Two (Fast-Paced Long Intervals)
• 4 minutes hard at 28–30spm / 4 minutes rest. Repeat five times. Your RPE for the hard section should be 8–9 out of 10.
• Resistance routine 1 (if possible, increase your weights).

Day Three
• Complete rest.

Day Four (Slow-Paced Long Row)
• 40 minutes at 18–22spm. Your RPE for this session should be 6–7 out of 10.

Day Five (Short-Paced Short Intervals)
• 1 minute hard at 30–32spm / 1 minute easy at 18–22spm. Repeat eight times. Your RPE for the hard section should be 8–9 out of 10.

Day Six (Active Rest)
• Spend 45–60 minutes doing any other activity or sport, apart from indoor rowing.
• Resistance routine 2 (if possible, increase your weights).

Day Seven
• Complete rest.

Week Eight
Day One (Steady-Paced Medium Row)
• 25 minutes at 24–26spm. Your RPE for the session should be 7–8 out of 10.

Day Two (Fast-Paced Long Intervals)
• 4 minutes hard at 28–30spm / 4 minutes rest. Repeat six times. Your RPE for the hard section should be 8–9 out of 10.
• Resistance routine 1.

Day Three
• Complete rest.

Day Four (Slow-Paced Long Row)
• 45 minutes at 18–22spm. Your RPE for this session should be 6–7 out of 10.

Day Five (Short Paced Short Intervals)
• 1 minute hard at 30–32spm / 1 minute easy at 18–22spm. Repeat eight times. Your RPE for the hard section should be 8–9 out of 10.

Day Six (Active Rest)
• Spend 45–60 minutes doing any other activity or sport, apart from indoor rowing.
• Resistance routine 2.

Day Seven
• Complete rest.

9 Indoor Rowing for Other Sports

Cross-Training

Even though the indoor rowing machine was originally designed to help amateur and professional outdoor rowers get the most out of training in the long winter months, it can still be very beneficial as a cross-training session within the normal training routine for your chosen sport. It has long been agreed that cross-training is vital, since it will help reduce the risk of injury, create muscular balance in your body, and help you perform better in your chosen sport. No matter what that may be, you will always run the risk of a repetitive strain injury, since you are constantly using the same muscles and repeating the same movement over again for training and competition. A simple change to your normal fitness routine by including some cross-training sessions on an indoor rowing machine will help to combat this problem. It will recruit a variety of muscle groups, including all the larger muscles, and help to improve overall aerobic conditioning, as well as higher intensity anaerobic workouts. It is a low-impact and non-jarring activity, which makes it safe and effective for the user. With the added bonus that you can track any improvement using the performance monitor, the indoor rowing machine is a great way to add variety to your sport's current fitness programme.

Running

Whether you are training for a sprint race on the track or a marathon on the road, it is always important to include some sort of speed work into your training routine if you want to improve your distances and times. Due to the high-impact nature of the sport of running, not every athlete or fitness enthusiast likes to continue their speed work sessions as running, since they are already clocking up a lot of time on their feet. This is where the indoor rowing machine is a good choice. It is an excellent means of gaining all the benefits of speed work without the high impact. When it comes to using such equipment for running, workouts can be easily transferred from the sport, since it takes approximately the same time to run the same distance you would cover on an indoor rowing machine. For running, the workout goal on an indoor rowing machine is to simulate a speed work session that might be done on the athletics track, without the high impact and constant pounding through the joints. The following workouts are based on some of the common running distances.

Sprint Distance (100m/200m/400m)
- Row easily for 5–10 minutes at 20–24spm to warm up.
- Row hard at 30–35spm and then row easy for recovery at 18–20spm.
Round 1: Hard 60 seconds / Easy 60 seconds.
Round 2: Hard 45 seconds / Easy 45 seconds.
Round 3: Hard 30 seconds / Easy 30 seconds.
Round 4: Hard 15 seconds / Easy 15 seconds.
Round 5: Hard 60 seconds.
- Row easily for 5–10 minutes at 18–20spm to cool down.

Middle Distance (800m/1500m)
- Row easily for 5–10 minutes at 20–24spm to warm up.
- Row hard at 28–35spm and then have a complete rest for a few minutes.
Round 1: Hard 4 minutes / Rest 2 minutes.
Round 2: Hard 3 minutes / Rest 3 minutes.
Round 3: Hard 2 minutes / Rest 4 minute.
(Repeat the above 3 rounds again).
- Row easily for 5–10 minutes at 18–20spm to cool down.

Long Distance (5,000m/10,000m/Half Marathon/Marathon)
- Row easily for 5–10 minutes at 20–24spm to warm up.
- Row hard for 25–30spm, making sure to up the pace to 30–35spm on the last 15 seconds of every 2 minutes and then have a complete rest.
Round 1: Hard 6 minutes / Rest 3 minutes.
Round 2: Hard 6 minutes / Rest 3 minutes.
Round 3: Hard 6 minutes.
Rest for 5–10 minutes and then repeat the above three rounds.
- Row easily for 5–10 minutes at 18–20spm to cool down.

Cycling

Every cyclist will have favourite hills they like to climb. You can design your indoor rowing workouts to prepare you for the climbs that you encounter on your cycling routes. For cycling, the workout goal on the indoor rowing machine is to simulate a serious of hill climbs.

- Row easily for 5–10 minutes at 20–24spm to warm up.
- Row at a steady pace at 25–28spm with 10-second fast bursts every minute at 30–35spm. After each round, row easy for recovery at 18–20spm.

Round 1: Steady 8 minutes with 10-second fast bursts / Easy 2 minutes.
Round 2: Steady 6 minutes with 10-second fast bursts / Easy 2 minutes.
Round 3: Steady 4 minutes with 10-second fast bursts / Easy 2 minutes.
Round 4: Steady 2 minutes with 10-second fast bursts / Easy 2 minutes.
- Row easily for 5–10 minutes at 18–20spm to cool down.

Hiking

Hiking as a fitness pastime or sport is generally a long steady workout that varies in intensity depending on the incline of the terrain. If your hike is taking you up a mountain then the intensity of the walk will usually build as you get higher, due to the steeper climb to reach the summit. Many hikers often carry a backpack, which requires good upper body strength as well as core strength. Indoor rowing is excellent for your cross-training because, as well as improving your endurance for the hike, it will help to strengthen your upper body and core for the added weight of your backpack. Most hikes start with the climb and finish with the descent. Even though the climb is usually tougher, the hike back down is what often leaves your body sore, owing to the eccentric leg contractions as you descend. The workout goal is to prepare your body for a long hike on mixed terrain of moderate-to-steep intensity.

- Row easily for 5–10 minutes at 20–24spm to warm up.
- Row three different intensities for each round (easy at 20–25spm, moderate at 25–30spm and hard at 30–35spm), before having a complete rest before the next round.
Round 1: Easy 8 minutes / Moderate 4 minutes / Hard 1 minute / Rest 2 minutes.
Round 2: Easy 6 minutes / Moderate 3

minutes / Hard 1 minute / Rest 2 minutes. Round 3: Easy 4 minutes / Moderate 2 minutes / Hard 1 minute / Rest 2 minutes.
• Row easily for 5–10 minutes at 18–20spm to cool down.

Rock Climbing and Bouldering

Rock climbing and bouldering is a sport that involves a series of intense, short cardio intervals. The length of the interval can vary depending on the length of the climb, as well as your skill and strength, but most rock climbers should prepare their body for intervals of 15 seconds up to as long as 5 minutes. Upper body strength and flexibility is also crucial for successful rock climbing and bouldering. Indoor rowing will not only help to improve your upper body strength and flexibility, but it will also prepare your body for the short cardio intervals involved with the sport.

• Row easily for 5–10 minutes at 20–24spm to warm up.
• Pyramid session involving rowing hard at 30–35spm and then rowing easy as a recovery at 18–20spm.
  Round 1: Hard 15 seconds / Easy 1 minute.
  Round 2: Hard 30 seconds / Easy 1 minute.
  Round 3: Hard 1 minute / Easy 1 minute.
  Round 4: Hard 2 minutes / Easy 1 minute.
  Round 5: Hard 4 minutes / Easy 1 minute.
  Round 6: Hard 2 minutes / Easy 1 minute.
  Round 7: Hard 1 minute / Easy 1 minute.
  Round 8: Hard 30 seconds / Easy 1 minute.
  Round 9: Hard 15 seconds.
  • Row easily for 5–10 minutes at 18–20spm to cool down.

Triathlon

A triathlon usually consists of a swim, followed by a cycle and finally a run, but there are many variations of triathlons, including some indoor competitions that have rowing as one of the three disciplines. Even if rowing is not one of your disciplines, the indoor rowing machine can be an excellent substitute for any of the other legs (the swim, bike or run). Generally the transition from the cycle to the run is the hardest, so when it comes to substituting the indoor rowing machine into your workouts it might be more beneficial to create a row-then-run combination if you are training for a standard outdoor triathlon, as it will help your body get used to the feeling of heavy legs before the run. The indoor rowing workout is designed not only to improve your fitness for the race, but also to practice for the cycle-to-run transition.

• Row easily for 5–10 minutes at 20–24spm to warm up.
• Row at a moderate intensity of 25–30spm and then move on to a short time on another triathlon discipline. Round 1: Moderate row 6–10 minutes / Get on the bike for a hard 3 minutes. Round 2:– Moderate row 6–10 minutes / Get on the treadmill for a hard 3 minutes. Have a complete rest of 5–10 minutes and then repeat both rounds again.
• Row easily for 5–10 minutes at 18–20spm to cool down.

Rugby and Football

Rugby and football players now need whole body aerobic fitness and strength to perform to their best on match day every week. The indoor rowing machine is excellent for this because it helps strengthen both upper and lower body as it improves overall cardiovascular fitness. The goal of the indoor rowing session is to simulate not only the steady endurance required to complete a full match, but also to get the body used to the random speed intervals that will occur throughout a game.

• Row for 5–10 minutes at 20–24spm to warm up.

- The session will move between a steady row section at 22–26spm and an interval session where you are rowing hard at 30–35spm.
  Round 1: Steady 5 minutes.
  Round 2: Hard 500m / Steady 500m. Repeat three times.
  Round 3: Steady 5 minutes.
  Round 4: Hard 300m / Steady 300m. Repeat four times.
  Round 5: Steady 5 minutes.
  Round 6: Hard 100m / Steady 100m. Repeat five times.
- Row easily for 5–10 minutes at 18–20spm to cool down.

Boxing and Mixed Martial Arts

Boxing has always been a popular sport, but mixed martial arts (MMA) is slowly becoming one of the most accepted contact sports in the world today. Both sports require a high level of fitness and total body strength. The indoor rowing machine is a great way to increase your fitness for the ring, as well as help improve the explosive power of many of the muscles used to both punch and kick. The workout goal is to improve your explosive power and overall cardiovascular fitness for a competition fight.

Boxing
- Row easily for 5–10 minutes at 20–24spm to warm up.
- Alternate between rowing hard at 30–35spm and rowing easy at 18–20spm.
  Round 1: Hard 15 seconds / Easy 15 seconds. Repeat for 3 minutes.
  Rest for 1 minute.
  Round 2: Hard 30 seconds / Easy 30 seconds. Repeat for 3 minutes.
  Rest for 1 minute.
  Repeat the above two rounds two or three times.
- Row easily for 5–10 minutes at 18–20spm to cool down.

MMA
- Row easily for 5–10 minutes at 20–24spm to warm up.
- Alternate between rowing hard at 30–35spm and rowing easy at 18–20spm.
  Round 1: Hard 15 seconds / Easy 15 seconds. Repeat for 2 minutes.
  Round 2: Hard 1 minute.
  Round 3: Hard 15 seconds / Easy 15 seconds). Repeat for 1 minute.
  Round 4: Hard 1 minute and then rest for 1 minute. Repeat the above rounds five times.
- Row easily for 5–10 minutes at 18–20spm to cool down.

Tennis, Squash and Badminton

Any type of racquet sport requires good speed and agility with a high level of cardiovascular fitness. More importantly, though, each sport involves random intervals at different intensities and times. The goal of the indoor rowing session is to simulate the random intervals that you would experience on the court during a match.

- Row easily for 5–10 minutes at 20–24spm to warm up.
- Alternate between rowing at a hard level at 30–35spm, a moderate level at 28–32spm and an easy level at 24–28spm.
  Round 1: Easy 30 seconds / Moderate 30 seconds / Hard 30 seconds. Repeat three times.
  Round 2: Easy 20 seconds / Moderate 30 seconds / Hard 40 seconds. Repeat three times.
  Round 3: Easy 30 seconds / Moderate 40 seconds / Hard 20 seconds. Repeat three times.
  Round 4: Easy 40 seconds / Moderate 20 seconds / Hard 30 seconds. Repeat three times.
  Round 5: Easy 30 seconds / Moderate 30 seconds / Hard 30 seconds. Repeat three times.
- Row easily for 5–10 minutes at 18–20spm to cool down.

10 Training

How It All Started

One of the main problems with training at home, or even in a health club, can be the lack of competition and support. Indoor rowing enthusiasts throughout the world decided to combat this common problem by setting up indoor rowing competitions. Two major figures in rowing have remained strong supporters of these events: the Amateur Rowing Association and the CRASH-B (Charles River All Star Has-Beens) rowing club. When it was first created, the indoor rowing race was five miles on a Concept2 Model A ergometer, but the introduction in 1986 of the Model B ergometer, with its new digital performance monitor display, led to the big race becoming 2,500m. The distance then changed again to meet the specific training demands of international coaches who were demanding 6,000m and 2,000m rankings during the winter training months. The current competition distance is 2,000m, a distance that was first organized by the C.R.A.S.H.-B. rowing club.

C.R.A.S.H.-B.

C.R.A.S.H.-B. originally comprised a group of 1970s US Olympic and World Team athletes who would rarely practice before a race, but most importantly, they all had a

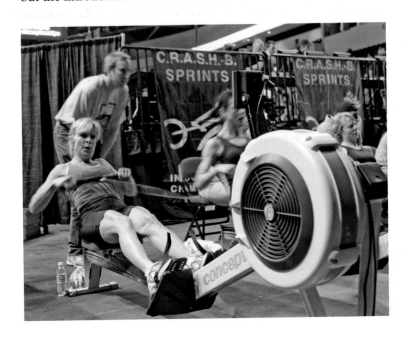

Indoor competitions are becoming more popular every year. (© Concept2)

great time doing it. The fun part of racing was definitely in their blood. In response to the US boycott of the Moscow Olympics in 1980, they started something new and exciting throughout the rowing world. It just so happened that around that time Concept2 had invented their Model A rower – the one with the bicycle wheel and the wooden handle. The C.R.A.S.H.-B. rowing enthusiasts were determined to break up the boredom of training in the long, cold winter months. They decided to organize a fun indoor regatta for around twenty rowers in Harvard's Newell Boathouse. As the years passed, C.R.A.S.H.-B.'s event slowly developed into what is now known as the International World Indoor Rowing Championships. The regatta moved on from Newell Boathouse and was held for many years at MIT's Rockwell Cage. In 1995 the regatta was moved to Harvard's Indoor Track Facility, which was around three times the size of Rockwell Cage. Since the demand was even greater than expected, in 1997 the C.R.A.S.H.-B. World Indoor Rowing Championships had to be moved to an even larger, more modern facility, the Reggie Lewis Track and Athletic Centre at Roxbury Community College. Since 2008 the International World Indoor Rowing Championships have been held at Boston University's Agganis Arena, a little downstream from C.R.A.S.H.-B.'s original site. The race is currently rowed on the latest Concept2 ergometers, as used by athletes and national teams and installed in universities, clubs and schools worldwide.

British Indoor Rowing Championships (BIRC)

The popularity of these championships has encouraged many other countries throughout Europe and Asia to get involved and organize their own annual competitions, including the English, Scottish, Welsh, Irish and Northern Irish championships. The British Indoor Rowing Championships, organized by Concept2, is one of the biggest indoor rowing events on the annual racing calendar and the largest indoor rowing event in the UK, with more than 3,000 entrants. The first British event was held in Henley-on-Thames in 1991, but continued to grow in subsequent years and since 2000 it has been held at the National Indoor Arena in Birmingham.

The standard race distance on indoor rowing machines, including for all competitions, is recognized worldwide as 2,000m. Covering this distance is very challenging. It is important to understand how to build up your training both safely and effectively, making sure that you get the most out of your body on race day. If you do not approach your training in a balanced and structured way, then you are only setting yourself up for disappointment. Regardless of whether you are at an Olympic level or a beginner, you need to be serious about your training build-up and give yourself at least eight weeks of solid training before a race. The more time you allow for training before the race, the more prepared you will be for the competition. If you find yourself with less than eight weeks to prepare, then I would recommend that you do not go ahead with the race, especially if you are new to training.

The Indoor Rowing Competition

The main indoor rowing season takes place during the winter months, usually starting around November and ending in March (many of the individual competition dates will vary each year). Now that indoor rowing has become more popular as a sport, you will not have to look too far to find a competition near you. The list overleaf shows some of the main 2000m indoor rowing competitions held throughout the year.

Competition	Month
British Indoor Rowing Championships	November
Irish Championships	December
European Championships	January
Scottish Championships	January
Welsh Championships	January
English Championships	February
World Indoor Rowing Championships	March

Indoor rowing competitions, depending on their size, will be judged on many different age categories, as well as two weight categories: lightweight and heavyweight. For men to qualify for the lightweight category they need to be 75kg or lighter on race day; anything over 75kg on race day will be classed as heavyweight. For women to qualify into the lightweight category they need to be 61.5kg or lighter; anything over 61.5kg on race day will be classed as heavyweight. Smaller competitions with fewer participants will usually be judged by using a handicapping system in order to make the competition as fair as possible for all competitors, since age and weight can both be factors influencing one's 2,000m indoor rowing time. According to Concept2, fitness performance in men declines at 0.12 per cent each year between the ages of 26 and 55, and at 0.83 per cent a year from age 56 onwards. Fitness performance in women decline at 0.23 per cent per year from the ages of 26 to 55 and at 0.74 per cent a year from age 56 onwards.

Detailed preset training programmes for different fitness level categories are presented in the appendix.

Marathon Training

Marathon training on the rower is not something you should consider lightly. The distance for the full marathon is 42,195m and the distance for the half-marathon is 21,097m. Each year the indoor rowing marathon and half-marathon distance is becoming more popular; there is even an annual marathon day that coincides with the London Marathon every April, organized by Concept2.

Training for the marathon on an indoor rowing machine is tough and the distances are long, but the good news is that the feeling of achievement you get at the end is definitely worth it. Preparations for a marathon take a lot of commitment. You should already have a good fitness level to work from. It is advisable to allow yourself four to five months to build up the distances required on an indoor rowing machine and prepare properly, not including the earlier base training of one to two months. If you decide to reduce your training time for an indoor rowing marathon, you will run a serious risk of not completing the distance on race day, since your body will not be accustomed to long times on the indoor rowing machine. Training for an indoor rowing marathon varies slightly from running a marathon, due to its low-impact nature. Because running is such a high-impact sport, there are important constraints that have to be made to your marathon training programme as the mileage and intensity start to increase, in order to make sure you minimize any risk of injury. However, when it comes to indoor rowing, some of these constraints can be relaxed slightly when you start to increase the distance and intensities due to its low-impact nature.

Before starting out with a marathon training programme, it is important to have spent some time on steady base training, alternating between an easy week and a tougher week to reduce the risk of over-training and injury. For two to three months, before you start to follow the marathon training build-up programme, you should be able to row between the accompanying two weekly sessions.

Marathon Paces

The marathon training plans for beginner, intermediate and advanced individuals (*see* Appendix) will make use of different paces and intensities, so before you attempt to follow one of the programmes it is recom-mended that you have had at least three months of regular training on an indoor rowing machine and have done time trials over 5,000m and 10,000m. Once you have completed those time trials, you can then predict your half-marathon pace and marathon pace. Calculating your paces for

each individual indoor rowing session in the programme is crucial to prevent over-training, as well as enabling you to hold back so that you can complete the longer distances required throughout the programme.

If you have not yet established a time for your 5,000m, 10,000m, half-marathon and marathon pace, you can work them out using the following simple formula: take your 500m pace for your latest 5,000m time trial and your 500m pace for your latest 10,000m time trail and calculate the difference. Then add the difference between your 500m paces at 5,000m and 10,000m to your 500m pace for 10,000m and this will give you an approximate 500m pace for the half marathon. You should then add twice this difference to your likely 500m pace for the half marathon pace to give your likely 500m pace for the full marathon. For example, if your 500m pace for 5,000m and 10,000m are 1:51 and 1:53 respectively, then the difference is two seconds. Your predicted half marathon 500m pace will be 1:55 and your predicted marathon 500m pace will be 1:59. Remember, though, that paces for each of the distances calculated in this way are to be used only for guidance, since how one

---

Marathon Training Weekly Sessions (A): The Easy Week

Day 1	Day 2	Day 3	Day 4	Day 5	Day 6	Day 7
2–3km (approx. 10–20min)	3–5km (approx. 15–30min)	Day off	2–3km (approx. 10–20min)	3–5km (approx. 15–30min)	Day off	Day off

Marathon Training Weekly Sessions (B): The Hard Week

Day 1	Day 2	Day 3	Day 4	Day 5	Day 6	Day 7
2–3km (approx. 10–20min)	3–5km (approx. 15–30min)	2–3km (approx. 10–20min)	3–5km (approx. 15–30min)	Day off	2–3km (approx. 10–20min)	6–10km (approx. 30–45min)

feels can make a big difference during the longer rowing sessions. As you follow your chosen marathon programme, the times in which you find yourself completing the long weekly row will give you a better feel for how accurate your original estimate is and you can adjust accordingly.

The Essential Long Row Session

When it comes to marathon training, by far the most important weekly row you will ever do is the long and slower-paced row. If the race you are training for requires a long row, you need to ensure you are preparing your body for precisely that. Make sure that there is a progressive build-up to the long rows throughout your training schedule, peaking as the race gets closer. One of the biggest mistakes many people make is to reach their peak too soon, which can have a negative effect on race day. The main benefits of the long weekly row are that it will train your body to produce energy from both your glycogen and fat stores. If you use all your glycogen too early, your body will experience what is commonly known as 'hitting the wall', where your body shut downs and you will find it close to impossible to continue. The long row allows you to try different hydration drinks, as well as help you work out the best way for you to take on the essential hydration needed during a marathon. The long row will also allow you to test different foods before the row, as well as the best time to eat them.

Detailed preset marathon training programmes for different fitness level categories are presented in the appendix.

11 Create Your Own Programme

When designing and planning your own indoor rowing programme, it is important firstly to understand the different training seasons and periodization. When you regularly train and work out you put your body under a form of stress. If you train correctly and safely, your body will eventually adapt to the stress under which you put it, making you fitter and stronger, as well as helping to change your body shape in the process. However, if you train incorrectly, working out on a regular basis can slow you down and make you feel weaker, sick, injured and demotivated. When you feel like this your performance is affected and you will not achieve your best. Therefore it is essential that you organize your training in a methodical way with the aim of creating a healthy balance between working out and letting your body recover. To help you achieve this balance, training can be broken down into different phases. This process is called periodization. For many fitness enthusiasts and athletes, the longest and most logical training period is usually planned out over a year – this is where your goals become important and you know what it is you're training for. One year can then be divided up into three further categories (athletes may refer to them as seasons):

• Off-season (base work)
• Pre-season (speed work)
• In-season (the taper)

The Phases

When fitness enthusiasts or athletes train through their off-season, they concentrate on longer indoor rowing sessions to build aerobic and muscular endurance, weight training to help with their strength and power, as well as cross-training on other sports or activities to minimize the risk of injury. During this phase your training is mostly broken down into what is known as base training. Base training can last as long as five months, but is usually six to twelve weeks. It really depends on how much time you have before your goal date or race date, as well as how fit you are before you start your base work. During the base work section you would normally do long-duration workouts on an indoor rowing machine at a low intensity. This base work section is intended to help you improve your aerobic and muscular endurance. As the base work training progresses, you will find that your tolerance of exercising on the indoor rowing machine will improve, enabling you to recover more quickly between each of your workouts. The base work section will give you the endurance you need to cope with the increase in intensity that will follow later in your programme. Some individuals put too much effort and intensity into the base work section, though, leaving them feeling exhausted by the time they reach the next phase, which will include more

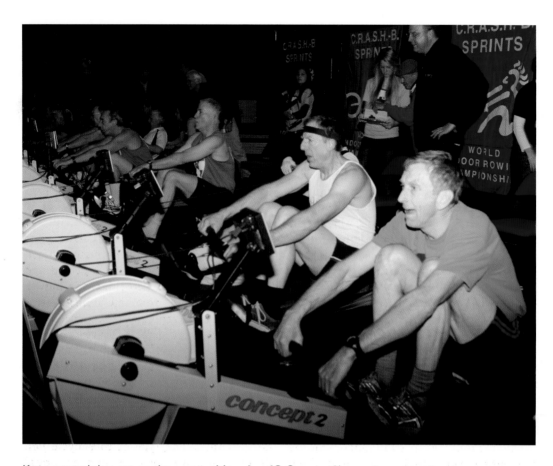

Keep your sights set on the competition day. (© Concept2)

speed work sessions. Stay patient, since speed work is a critical section in any indoor rowing programme.

After you have successfully completed your base work section, you are now ready to move on to what is known as the speed work section. This section usually takes four to eight weeks, again depending on the timeframe of your goal. Time spent in this section is very important because this is where you will make most of your performance gains. If done correctly, you should be decreasing your training volume, but increasing your training intensity. As before, your body will slowly adapt to the stress you are putting it

under, resulting in you becoming faster. It is important to remember, though, that if you increase the intensity too much and too soon it will only result in you overtraining. This is why you should try to give yourself more rest or active recovery (cross-training on another sport or activity) between each of your speed work sessions. Due to the intensity of speed work sessions, try to mix in one or two endurance-based longer sessions each week.

Tapering is crucial if you are training for an indoor rowing event or competition, ensuring that you are at your strongest on race day. The longer the race, and the more important it is to you, the longer you should take to gradually reduce your training volume. A common mistake made during the tapering section is to cut back on your training intensity too soon. You should only reduce the intensity in the final couple of days before the race. Even though you can reduce your training volume anywhere up to two weeks before your race, depending on the race length, your training intensity in each session should remain constant. When you keep your indoor rowing session intensity constant, you will be more fully aware of the intensity you should give on race day. Remember, though, that tapering is a very personal thing and what works for one person may not for another, so you should experiment and see what suits you. Tapering should generally take between two and fourteen days – reducing the workout volume approximately two weeks before the race and reducing the workout intensity two to three days before race day.

Training Cycles

When planning your own indoor rowing programme you should also think about training cycles, or the tough sections and easy sections of your training programme. If you try to make every single indoor rowing session as tough as possible, you will only be setting yourself up for disappointment and complete exhaustion. There are three main different types of training cycles: microcycles (day to day), mesocycles (week to week) and macrocycles (year to year).

Microcycle

A microcycle is used to maximize your workout time each day by trying to give each of your indoor rowing workouts a balance. If planned properly, you will allow yourself to recover between each session: the more recovery you allow yourself between indoor rowing workouts, the more effective they become and the more progress you will make. One of the easiest ways to provide this balance to your workouts is to use the easy/hard approach to training, alternating between an easy workout one day and a hard workout on the next. The easy days can be a drop in workout volume or intensity, or, if you prefer, you can have a complete rest from training.

Mesocycle

A mesocycle is used to maximize your training on a week-to-week basis. It will have a built-in recovery period to compensate for the more intense indoor rowing training you may experience during your programme. Mesocycles are something that should occur on a regular basis throughout your training programme, allowing you to recover with an easy week between every two and six weeks to help you stay away from the severe training fatigue that can wear you down and destroy your indoor rowing performance. The type of mesocycle you design will come down to your individual preference, as well as the intensity of your training. If in doubt, start by alternating between an easy week's training and a tougher week. As your indoor rowing experience increases, you can then change your mesocycle rest week to every three or four training weeks throughout your training programme. Learn to listen to your body; it will let you know when you need to rest.

Macrocycle

A macrocycle is used by people who want to create a balance with their indoor rowing training over the course of a year. The macrocycle is important when you have a future goal or a variety of races you need to prepare for throughout the year. Based on your future events, you should then break down your year into the three main categories mentioned above: off-season, pre-season and in-season. The macrocycle is usually the first cycle you should plan out. Once this is fixed you can then move on to planning the mesocycle (week-to-week) and microcycle (day-to-day) details of your indoor rowing sessions.

Structuring a Training Programme

When it comes to structuring your indoor rowing training programme, the key is to keep training sessions that are similar in intensity well apart from each other. In other words, do not do three days of nothing but high-intensity interval speed work. This goes back to the earlier comments about planning microcycles and alternating between easy training days and tougher training days. If you are able to keep workouts of similar intensity apart, it will help you recover and so perform better in future sessions. In short, it will make you fitter and stronger.

Top Mistakes When Designing a Programme

Too much effort during your base work section. Base training is designed to help your recovery rate and improve your tolerance to training, preparing your body for the upcoming speed work section of your indoor rowing training programme. Base work is not there to make you go faster. Save that for the speed work.

Too much speed work. Speed work is something that does not need to be done every single day, because doing so will only result in you burning out during indoor rowing sessions. If you want to get the best results possible from speed work, and depending on your experience, speed work should be done two (beginners), three (intermediate) or four (advanced) times a week.

Reducing your training intensity during the taper. If you want to race your best in competition, you have to decrease your total training volumes a few weeks before the race. That does not mean, however, that you have to slow down as well. You should keep up your speed work intensity, even though distances and times may be reduced. If you stop working on your speed at this stage of your programme, then you will run the risk of your body quickly losing all the speed work you worked so hard to achieve. To stay fast on race day, make sure to keep some sort of speed sessions throughout the taper section and only reduce the intensity of your workouts for a couple of days before the big event.

Programme Design
Beginner

You should ideally adopt the following programme layout if you are new to indoor rowing as a sport, new to fitness, or have only trained for one to two days a week for the past few months.

Microcycle

Day 1	Day 2	Day 3	Day 4	Day 5	Day 6	Day 7	Repeat...
Hard	Easy	Hard	Easy	Hard	Easy	Easy	Repeat...

Mesocycle

Week 1	Week 2	Week 3	Week 4	Week 5	Week 6	Repeat...
Hard	Easy	Hard	Easy	Hard	Easy	Repeat...

Macrocycle

Month 1	Month 2	Month 3	Month 4	Month 5	Month 6
Base work	Base work	Base work	Base work	Base work	Base work

Month 7	Month 8	Month 9	Month 10	Month 11	Month 12
Base work	Base work	Speed work	Speed work	Speed work	Taper and race

Intermediate

You should follow the programme layout for intermediates if you have used an indoor rowing machine in your workouts and have been training regularly for two to four days a week for six months to a year.

Microcycle

Day 1	Day 2	Day 3	Day 4	Day 5	Day 6	Day 7	Repeat...
Easy	Moderate	Hard	Easy	Moderate	Hard	Easy	Repeat...

Mesocycle

Week 1	Week 2	Week 3	Week 4	Week 5	Week 6	Repeat...
Hard	Hard	Easy	Hard	Hard	Easy	Repeat...

Macrocycle

Month 1	Month 2	Month 3	Month 4	Month 5	Month 6
Base work	Base work	Base work	Base work	Base work	Base work

Month 7	Month 8	Month 9	Month 10	Month 11	Month 12
Base work	Speed work	Speed work	Speed work	Speed work	Taper and race

Advanced

You should follow this programme layout if you have used an indoor rowing machine on a regular basis within your workouts and have trained regularly for four days or more for over a year.

Microcycle

Day 1	Day 2	Day 3	Day 4	Day 5	Day 6	Day 7	Repeat...
Easy	Hard	Hard	Easy	Hard	Hard	Easy	Repeat...

Mesocycle

Week 1	Week 2	Week 3	Week 4	Etc.
Hard	Hard	Hard	Easy	Etc.

Macrocycle

Month 1	Month 2	Month 3	Month 4	Month 5	Month 6
Base work	Base work	Base work	Base work	Base work	Base work

Month 7	Month 8	Month 9	Month 10	Month 11	Month 12
Speed work	Speed work	Speed work	Speed work	Speed work	Taper and race

12 Good Nutrition

The purpose of this chapter is not to describe the latest diet fad, or show you how to create your own perfect individual nutrition programme. It is about educating you in the basics involved for a balanced, healthy diet. In order to stay healthy your diet must contain adequate amounts of all the essential nutrients: carbohydrates, proteins, fats, water, vitamins and minerals. If you lack any of the essential nutrients, it will have a negative effect on your indoor rowing workouts, not to mention your race day performance if you enter a competition. To check that you are getting a good balance of nutritious foods on a daily basis, it is a good idea to follow a basic food pyramid, a concept designed to meet the nutritional needs of any individual who performs regular exercise. The foods in the lower level of the pyramid should form the main part of your daily diet, while those foods towards the top of the pyramid should be eaten in smaller quantities.

Food Pyramid Levels

Bottom Level

The bottom level of the food pyramid provides the biggest percentage of your daily calories and should consist of fruit and vegetables, as well as wholegrain foods. The fruit and vegetables section of the bottom level (5–9 portions a day – one portion can approximately fit in your palm) should contain essential vitamins, minerals, antioxidants and fibre, which are vital for optimal health and workout performance. The whole-grain section (4–6 portions a day) can be found in foods like cereals, rice, pasta, bread, oats, beans, lentils and potatoes, which together supply your body with high levels of the long-lasting carbohydrate energy you will need to fuel your indoor rowing workouts.

Middle Level

The middle level includes two different sections, the calcium section and the protein section. The calcium section (2–4 portions a day) of the middle level is provided by a variety of dairy products, nuts, as well as pulses. The protein section (2–4 portions a day), should include lean meat, fish, poultry, eggs, soya or quorn. Beans, lentils and dairy products can also contribute towards your daily protein needs.

Top Level

The top level of the food pyramid should provide the lowest percentage of your daily calories, the fat section (1–2 portions a day). Everybody is frightened of eating fat in their diet, but the fact is that your body requires essential fats if you want to protect against heart disease, as well as improve your endurance and recovery. You can get these essential fats from nuts, seeds, olive oil, flax seed oil, sunflower oil and oily fish.

Essential Nutrients

Carbohydrates

Carbohydrates are known as the energy food. They can be divided up into two basic forms:

simple carbohydrates (sugars) and complex carbohydrates (starches and fibre). Simple carbohydrates comprise fast-releasing sugars that give you a quick energy boost, followed by a fast energy low – not ideal. Simple carbohydrates will usually look, taste and feel sweet and sticky, for example sugars, jams and sweets. On the other hand, complex carbohydrates will have slow-releasing sugars that supply your body with steady energy over a longer period of time. Complex carbo-hydrates are usually dense starchy foods, for example cereals, bread, pasta, rice, vegetables and potatoes – ideal for endurance-related sports like indoor rowing.

Taking on carbohydrates before an indoor rowing session can be an excellent way to give your body the boost it requires to perform the workout, but when it comes to eating before exercise, what is the best time to eat? Unfortunately there is no perfect answer, since the choice of pre-workout meals and snacks can vary from person to person. Generally, you should try to eat between two and four hours before training on an indoor rowing machine, leaving enough time for your stomach to settle so you feel comfortable during your workout. Some of the more popular pre-workout carbohydrate snacks, taken one or two hours before exercise, are fresh fruit, dried fruit, a smoothie, yoghurt or an energy bar. The more popular pre-workout carbohydrate meals, eaten two to four hours before exer-cise, are a jacket potato with beans, tuna or chicken, pasta with vegetables, mixed bean salad, wholegrain cereal, porridge, or a chicken salad sandwich.

People sometimes worry about taking on fuel during their workout, but if your training session is less than an hour long then taking anything other than water is unnecessary, providing your pre-workout food was good. If you are planning to work out for longer than an hour, though, you may need to consume more carbohydrates during exercise to maintain your blood sugar levels, allow you to exercise for longer and prevent you from burning out. Which foods are best? It makes sense that any food you take during exercise needs to be digested and absorbed quickly and easily by your body. That is why many people enjoy the ease of taking one of the many isotonic energy drinks available. Other foods can also be suitable, however, and among the most popular carbohydrate snacks taken during exercise are ripe bananas, raisins, fruit bars and energy gels. If you are training for an indoor rowing race that requires you to take carbohydrates during the session, for example a marathon, half-marathon or team relay, you need to make sure that you try a variety of foods to see what works best for you.

The length of time it takes for you to refuel your body after an indoor rowing session or race depends on the workout intensity, the amount of muscle damage and your training experience. The higher the intensity and length of your workout, the more energy your body will use, which determines how long your body will take to refuel. It can take anywhere from only twenty minutes to refuel from a short, intense interval workout up to a few days to refuel after a long session like a marathon. Muscle damage after training can be higher when certain activities like weight training are mixed in with your indoor rowing sessions, so it can take a few days after such a session to refuel your body and repair your muscle fibres. Your fitness experience can also be a major factor as to how long it takes your body to refuel after workouts and recover. The less experienced fitness enthusiast or athlete will take longer to refuel, which explains why experienced athletes can train every day, while less experienced individuals should give themselves plenty of rest between each training session. Some of the more popular post-workout snacks, taken within two hours after exercise, are a large portion of fresh fruit, yoghurt, sports bar, meal replacement shake, sandwich with lean meat and salad, and a selection of dried fruit and nuts, as well as wholegrain cereal with milk.

Protein

Protein is part of every cell and tissue in your body, including muscle tissue, internal organs, tendons, hair and nails. Protein is essential to help your body grow and repair itself. Many people still believe that protein is only important to individuals who concentrate their workout time on weight training, but intense endurance training, such as indoor rowing, can increase protein requirements because of the increased breakdown of protein during each training session. The additional protein in a healthy balanced diet is required to repair and recover the muscle tissue after endurance training. If you mix weight training with your sessions on an indoor rowing machine, however, your protein requirements are even more important due to the rate that protein is broken down in the muscles after resistance training.

Protein is made up of what are called amino acids. There are twenty different types of amino acids, twelve of which are categorized as non-essential amino acids because, if they are in short supply, your body can easily make them. The other eight are known as essential amino acids, since your body cannot make them. So although we need to eat protein on a daily basis to keep our cells topped up with amino acids, we need to pay attention to the sources of the essential ones. Individuals who regularly eat complete proteins from meat, or from animal produce such as eggs, milk and cheese, will have no problem in meeting their essential amino acid needs. Most plant proteins, however, lack one or two of the essential amino acids, so it may be necessary to ensure a mixed diet

with soy-bean products, cereals, legumes and nuts to give your body the essential amino acids it needs.

Be careful not to consume too much protein as excess protein and amino acids that your body does not need will be excreted with difficulty by the kidneys. This can sometimes lead to kidney stones, as well as to kidney damage.

Fat

Many people still believe that all fat is bad, but the fact is that our bodies need fat to function. A healthy amount of fat in our daily diet will help protect our internal organs, will be used for energy, help our growth development, and help in the uptake and storage of fat-soluble vitamins. The problem that most people run into, and the reason why fat gets such a bad press, is that we generally eat far too much fat in our daily diet, especially the wrong type of fat, and this can lead to obesity, heart disease and other problems. A diet that has less than 25 per cent of total fat on a regular basis would be classed as unhealthy. An early sign of deficiency would be a deterioration in skin and hair condition.

Once you have been able to reduce the total amount of fat in your diet, you then need to examine the types of fat in your diet. There are two main types of fat: saturated fat (mainly derived from animal sources and commonly solid at room temperature) and unsaturated fat (mainly derived from plant sources and tending to be liquid at room temperature). No more than 25 per cent of the total amount of fat consumed should be saturated fat, mainly since this carries with it high amounts of cholesterol, which can lead to heart disease. Certain of the unsaturated fats are essential to our body and also have beneficial effects on our blood and clotting factors. These include the omega-3 and omega-6 fatty acids, which are found in a number of different plant sources, such as evening primrose oil and rape seed oil, as well as fish oils. This is why it is important to eat oily fish regularly.

Vitamins

Vitamins are chemicals found naturally in food that are needed in small amounts for us to perform specific functions. There are two different classes of vitamins: water soluble (vitamin C and vitamin B group) and fat soluble (vitamin A, vitamin D, vitamin E and vitamin K). The water soluble vitamins are essential to help our body's chemical processes function properly, including the extraction of energy from food and the growth of new body tissues. The fat soluble vitamins have a more varied range of functions, but are equally as important: vitamin A is needed for vision, vitamin D is essential for bone growth and helps to regulate calcium levels in our body, vitamin K is important for blood clotting and vitamin E protects our body's tissues against chemical damage.

Although some of these vitamins, particularly the fat soluble ones, can be obtained from animal sources, the best way to ensure an adequate intake is to eat a wide variety of fruit and vegetables on a daily basis. In addition, there are some vitamins that may need to be taken in additional quantities in order to meet the recommended daily allowance for very active people. These so-called anti-oxidant vitamins –vitamins A, C and E – help to fight against the damaging effect of oxygen free radicals that build up in our bodies as a result of normal day-to-day activity.

Minerals

Minerals can fall into two main groups: macro elements, such as sodium, potassium and calcium, and trace elements, for example copper, zinc and iron. The list of trace elements is extensive and each of these metals is usually required in minute portions to perform specialist functions in our bodies. In the macro elements section there are a few minerals that we need in visible amounts – sodium and calcium. Although sodium has many functions in the body, the main one is that it helps to regulate our water balance. The problem with sodium, though, is that it dissolves easily in the blood and cannot be cleared from the blood into cells without some difficulty. The dissolved sodium makes blood a lot more concentrated than the fluid cells inside, which results in raising the amount of blood the heart has to pump around the body and leading to raised blood pressure. It is estimated that we regularly consume three to four times the recommended allowance of sodium each day, so look out for all the hidden salts in your foods. Calcium is essential for many functions of the body, including muscle contraction and nerve transmission. It is probably better known, though, as one of the main components of strong healthy bones. Calcium is crucial for many women due to the higher risk of osteoporosis in later life. Although calcium can be obtained from vegetarian sources, it is mainly found in dairy products such as milk and cheese, but since these products are also high in fat, many people decide to omit them from their diet, resulting in a lower calcium intake.

Water

Water is one of the most important nutrients your body will ever need, not least since about 60 per cent of our bodies is water. Water can serve many vital functions, including providing a transportation system for the body, moving nutrients, oxygen, vitamins and minerals to where they need to be, as well as moving waste products out. Water also plays a vital role in regulating our body temperature and provides the environment in which every chemical reaction in our body takes place.

A loss of 2 per cent body weight of water can seriously compromise your workout performance, while a loss of 5 per cent can be fatal. A human body suffers a loss of between two and three litres of water per day at rest and this has to be replaced if you do not want your workouts to suffer. If you exercise regularly, you may require an additional one or two litres of water per day, depending on the workout intensity and environment temperature. Some of the water we need will come from the food we eat. Fruit and vegetables contain a very high water content and it has been estimated that our recommended fruit and vegetable daily intake can supply between one and one-and-a-half litres of water a day. Bear in mind, though, that certain things you drink, such as coffee, tea, alcohol and many soft drinks, can make matters worse by accelerating the water loss from the body. It can sometimes be difficult to decide if and when you are dehydrated, but remember that thirst cannot be used as an indicator of your fluid status. Thirst is the first stage of dehydration, so by the time you feel thirsty it is already too late. It is also likely that when you drink water to rehydrate, your thirst will feel satisfied long before you have actually fully hydrated. The bottom line is that the best fluid to drink is water itself and the best approach is to drink regularly throughout the day.

13 Injuries and Their Prevention

Please note that none of the exercises mentioned in this chapter are intended for individuals to do while suffering with an injury. These exercises may, however, improve your overall flexibility and strength, therefore improving technique and leading to safer exercising, helping to reduce the risk of injury.

Due to the low-impact nature of indoor rowing, injuries should be rare if your technique is good, but as with any sport, there is always a small risk of injury. No matter how skilled or experienced an individual is, injury can pop up at any time, so it is important to be be knowledgeable about some of the most common injuries and problems – after all, you never know if and when it will happen to you.

Lower Back Pain

Lower back pain is probably one of the most common complaints among individuals who take up indoor rowing. Some may experience just a small nagging ache that does not affect them too much; others may suffer sharp pain that often makes daily tasks unbearable. If you experience back pain of any kind, you should stop exercising immediately. If the pain you feel is not relieved by rest, you should then seek the help of a registered medical professional.

Static Stretching Exercises to Reduce the Risk of Injury
Seated Spinal Twist

Start in a seated position on the floor, with both legs straight out in front of you. Bend one leg in and twist your upper body to the inside of that leg, placing the opposite arm on the outside of your bent leg and using your other arm behind you for support. Twist your body to the point of tension and hold for approximately thirty seconds before repeating on each side two to three times.

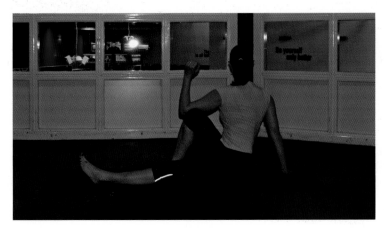

Twist until you feel tension for the seated spinal twist stretch.

Seated Cross Leg Reach

Start in a seated position on the floor with both legs crossed in front of you. Place both hands on the floor in front of your legs and slowly walk your hands out on the floor as you bend your body forward. Bend forward until you feel the point of tension and hold for approximately thirty seconds before repeating on each side for two to three times.

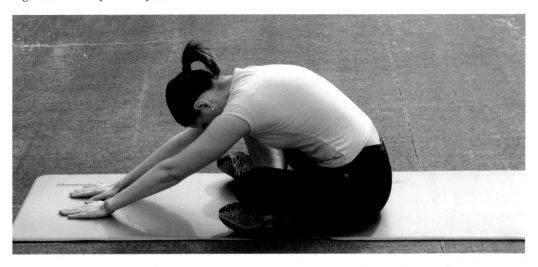

Slowly walk your hands forward for the seated cross leg stretch.

Strength Exercises to Reduce the Risk of Injury

Back Raise

Start by lying on your stomach. Place both hands on either side of your head and tuck your chin in. Slowly lift your chest up from the floor and return back down in a steady controlled movement, remembering to keep both feet on the floor throughout the move. Start by repeating the exercise for one set of ten repetitions, and slowly build it up to two sets of twenty repetitions.

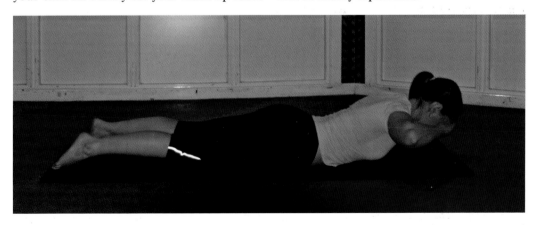

Keep both feet grounded during the back raise.

The Bridge

Start by lying on your back, with both feet on the floor and a bend on both knees. Keep your arms pressed down firmly on the floor, lift your hips up, squeeze your bottom and tense your stomach in the process, until your hips are in a straight line with your shoulders and knees. Start by repeating the exercise for one set of ten repetitions, and slowly build it up to two sets of twenty repetitions.

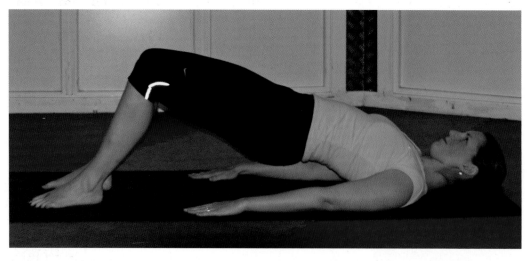

Remember to squeeze your buttocks at the top of the bridge.

Knee Pain

There are many causes and variations of knee pain, but when it comes to the sport of indoor rowing, one of the most common causes of knee pain is overuse (a repetitive strain injury). It is usually down to either rowing too many long workout sessions each week, or to tiredness or poor technique making your thigh muscles less efficient. Treatment for properly diagnosed overuse injuries is a simple process – initially you need to follow and apply the RICE (rest, ice, compression and elevation) principle for the specific injury. If the pain you feel is not relieved, you should then seek the help of a registered medical professional.

Static Stretching Exercises to Reduce the Risk of Injury

Standing Thigh Stretch
Start on your feet and slowing bring one foot

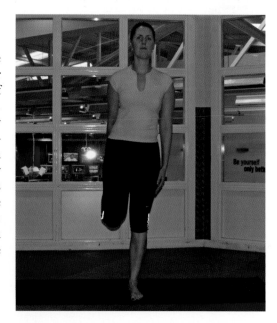

Keep both knees together for the standing thigh stretch.

up towards your bottom, holding on to the ankle. Bring your foot up to the point of tension and hold. Remember to keep both knees together throughout the stretch. Hold for approximately thirty seconds and repeat on each side two to three times.

Lying Back Double Thigh Stretch
Start on your knees, with your hands by your side on the floor. Slowly walk your hands behind as you lean your upper body backwards. Hold at the point of tension. Depending on how good your flexibility is, you might be able to lean back onto your forearms, or even all the way back until your back is on the floor. Remember, though, to take it slowly and do not go too far back too soon. Hold for approximately thirty seconds and repeat on each side two to three times.

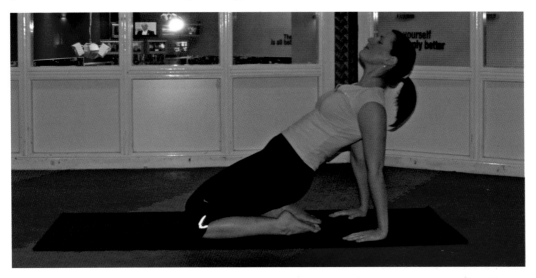

Lean back slowly for the lying back double thigh stretch.

Strength Exercises to Reduce the Risk of Injury
One-leg Squat
Start by getting your balance, standing on one leg. Slowly sit back, remembering to keep your chest high and bending your knee in line with your big toe and second toe. Sit back as low as your body will allow, but do not allow your hips to go lower than your knee; then return to the top. Start by repeating the exercise for one set of ten repetitions, and slowly build it up to two sets of twenty repetitions.

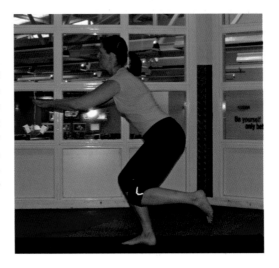

Keep your hips higher than your knee for the one leg squat.

119

Lunge

Start with one leg forward and one back, keeping both feet about hip width apart. With your chest high, bend your back knee and lower your whole body straight down until your knees are approximately at right angles, then return to the top. Remember not to lean forward, and keep your front knee in line with your big toe and second toe. Start by repeating the exercise for one set of ten repetitions and slowly build it up to two sets of twenty repetitions.

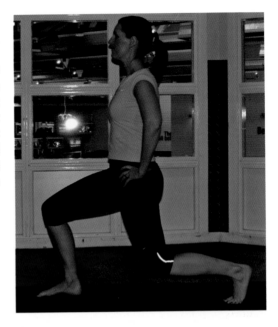

Be careful not to lean forward during the lunge.

Wrist Pain

When it comes to indoor rowing, the common symptoms of wrist injuries are as follows: pain, swelling, redness, a feeling of heat and weakness of the wrist, usually over the back surface. You would usually feel pain along the wrist with one specific movement or cocking of the wrist, but it is not uncommon for all movements to feel uncomfortable. If your wrist injury is not relieved by rest, the assessment from a registered medical professional should be sought.

Strength Exercises to Reduce the Risk of Injury

Stress Ball Squeeze

Holding a stress ball, or even a squash ball, start to squeeze the ball. Start by repeating the exercise for one set of ten repetitions, and slowly build it up to two sets of twenty repetitions.

Wrist Twists with a Weight

Holding on to a light dumbbell, slowing bend your wrist up and down, as well as twisting it from left and right. Start by repeating the exercise for one set of ten repetitions, and slowly build it up to two sets of twenty repetitions.

Other Problems

Overtraining

Overtraining can become very serious if left alone and not recognized. Constant tiredness, irritability, insomnia, decreased appetite and decreased training performance are all symptoms to look out for if you are training too much. To make sure that you do not fall into the trap of overtraining, you should always remember to rest between your workout sessions: it is important to recover both physically and mentally. If you get into the habit of having regular rest, you will be rewarded with increased enthusiasm, as well as better workout performances. One of the most common factors with all successful athletes and fitness enthusiasts appears to be that the

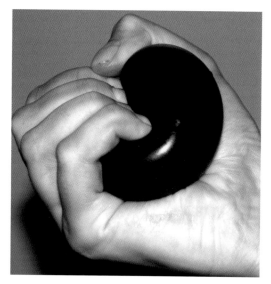 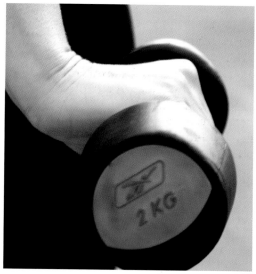

The stress ball squeeze is excellent for wrist injuries.

Move the weight in all directions in the wrist twist.

more they train, the better they will perform. However, performance and results depend not only on a high level of commitment, but also on a carefully designed programme where training is complemented with the appropriate recovery. Overtraining is still a very common phenomenon that affects many individuals, from the fitness enthusiast up to the sports professional, so it is important to recognize when it is happening and address it before it destroys your performance. While most athletes who become overtrained miss only a few days of training (if action is taken early), the symptoms can, and usually do, last much longer. This is particularly true for those who ignore the early warning signs.

Due to the long-term effects of overtraining, it is critical that you prevent yourself from overstepping the mark between pushing yourself beyond what you are capable of doing in workout sessions and overtraining – it can sometimes be a fine line. As this mark is often blurred and differs from person to person, pushing your fitness limits should only be done by individuals experienced in fitness training. If you are a complete novice to indoor rowing and fitness training, then you should never push yourself to that limit. Usually, you will never know that you are overtraining until it has happened, so remember that it is important to give yourself the appropriate rest days between your workouts and indoor rowing sessions, especially the tougher workouts.

Appendix

Training Programmes

2,000m Training Programmes

The following preset programmes are divided into three main fitness level categories: beginner, intermediate and advanced. Be careful when choosing your fitness category, because if you start too high you will find it difficult to stick to. Be honest with yourself on where you need to start, as well as how many sessions you can actually fit in each week. The workouts will be based on four different training intensities: aerobic low zone (Z-1) at 60–75% of your maximum heart rate, tempo low zone (Z-2) at 75–80% of your maximum heart rate, threshold medium zone (Z-3) at 80–95% of your maximum heart rate, and anaerobic high zone (Z-4) at 95–100% of your maximum heart rate.

Beginner Level. You should start at this level if you feel that you have done little to no exercise in the past six to twelve months, averaging zero to two sessions a week. This section will give you ten different programmes to choose from, starting with eight weeks to race day up to twenty-six weeks to race day. If you want to follow this beginner level section you need to commit yourself to work out for three to four sessions each week.

Intermediate Level. If you want to start at this level you should have been doing regular exercise over the past six to twelve months, averaging three sessions a week. This section will give you ten different programmes to choose from, starting with eight weeks to race day up to twenty-six weeks to race day. To follow this intermediate level section you need to commit yourself to work out for four to five sessions each week.

Advanced Level. You should start at this advanced level if you feel that you have been doing regular exercise in the past six to twelve months, averaging four to six sessions a week. This advanced level section will again give you ten different programmes to choose from, starting with eight weeks to race day up to twenty-six weeks to race day. To follow this section you need to commit yourself to work out for five to six sessions each week.

Beginner Programmes
Each of the beginner programmes will alternate between an easy training week and a hard training week, to make sure that you get the rest required to perform well and not overtrain. Session four of each week is an optional session, depending on whether or not you have the time that week to train three or four times. If the session involves intervals, you should give yourself the same time, if not a little more, to rest. For example, if a session requires you to row $2 \times$ 4 minutes, then you should give yourself a rest period of 4–5 minutes between each set. Each of the beginner programmes will include two time trials (2,000m test), one at the start of the programme and one halfway through. You should aim for your heart rate

to be in Z-3 up to as high as Z-4 (80–100% of your maximum heart rate) for each 2,000m time trial. Time trials are important to gauge how you are improving through the programme, as well as to give you an idea on how to perform on race day. Remember to warm up and cool down with every indoor rowing workout session.

8 Weeks

Week	Session 1	Session 2	Session 3	Session 4
1 (easy)	2,000m TEST	3 × 5min (Z-2)	10min (Z-1)	10min (Z-1)
2 (hard)	3 × 10min (Z-2)	5 × 5min (Z-2)	15min (Z-1)	15min (Z-1)
3 (easy)	2 × 10min (Z-2)	3 × 5min (Z-2)	15min (Z-1)	15min (Z-1)
4 (hard)	3 × 10min (Z-2)	5 × 5min (Z-2)	20min (Z-1)	20min (Z-1)
5 (easy)	2,000m Test	3 × 5min (Z-2)	20min (Z-1)	20min (Z-1)
6 (hard)	20 strokes hard, 20 strokes easy (repeat 6 times)	5 × 5min (Z-2)	30min (Z-1)	30min (Z-1)
7 (easy)	10 strokes hard, 20 strokes easy (repeat 6 times)	3 × 5min (Z-2)	20min (Z-1)	20min (Z-1)
8 (race week)	15min (Z-2)	10min (Z-2)	REST	RACE

10 Weeks

Week	Session 1	Session 2	Session 3	Session 4
1 (easy)	2000m TEST	3 × 5min (Z-2)	10min (Z-1)	10min (Z-1)
2 (hard)	3 × 10min (Z-2)	5 × 5min (Z-2)	15min (Z-1)	15min (Z-1)
3 (easy)	2 × 10min (Z-2)	3 × 5min (Z-2)	15min (Z-1)	15min (Z-1)
4 (hard)	3 × 10min (Z-2)	5 × 5min (Z-2)	20min (Z-1)	20min (Z-1)
5 (easy)	2 × 10min (Z-2)	3 × 5min (Z-2)	20min (Z-1)	20min (Z-1)
6 (hard)	2000m TEST	5 × 5min (Z-2)	30min (Z-1)	30min (Z-1)
7 (easy)	10 strokes hard, 20 strokes easy (repeat 6 times)	3 × 5min (Z-2)	30min (Z-1)	30min (Z-1)
8 (hard)	20 strokes hard, 20 strokes easy (repeat 6 times)	5 × 5min (Z-2)	30min (Z-1)	30min (Z-1)
9 (easy)	10 strokes hard, 20 strokes easy (repeat 6 times)	3 × 5min (Z-2)	20min (Z-1)	20min (Z-1)
10 (race week)	15min (Z-2)	10min (Z-2)	REST	RACE

12 Weeks

Week	Session 1	Session 2	Session 3	Session 4
1 (easy)	2,000m TEST	3 × 5min (Z-2)	10min (Z-1)	10min (Z-1)
2 (hard)	3 × 10min (Z-2)	5 × 5min (Z-2)	15min (Z-1)	15min (Z-1)
3 (easy)	2 × 10min (Z-2)	3 × 5min (Z-2)	15min (Z-1)	15min (Z-1)
4 (hard)	3 × 10min (Z-2)	5 × 5min (Z-2)	20min (Z-1)	20min (Z-1)
5 (easy)	2 × 10min (Z-2)	3 × 5min (Z-2)	20min (Z-1)	20min (Z-1)
6 (hard)	3 × 10min (Z-2)	5 × 5min (Z-2)	30min (Z-1)	30min (Z-1)
7 (easy)	2,000m TEST	3 × 5min (Z-2)	30min (Z-1)	30min (Z-1)
8 (hard)	20 strokes hard, 20 strokes easy (repeat 6 times)	5 × 5min (Z-2)	2 × 1,000m with 3–5min rest (Z-3)	30min (Z-1)
9 (easy)	10 strokes hard, 20 strokes easy (repeat 6 times)	3 × 5min (Z-2)	30min (Z-1)	30min (Z-1)
10 (hard)	20 strokes hard, 20 strokes easy (repeat 6 times)	5 × 5min (Z-2)	2 × 1,000m with 3–5min rest (Z-3)	30min (Z-1)
11 (easy)	10 strokes hard, 20 strokes easy (repeat 6 times)	3 × 5min (Z-2)	20min (Z-1)	20min (Z-1)
12 (race week)	15min (Z-2)	10min (Z-2)	REST	RACE

14 Weeks

Week	Session 1	Session 2	Session 3	Session 4
1 (easy)	2,000m TEST	3 × 5min (Z-2)	10min (Z-1)	10min (Z-1)
2 (hard)	3 × 10min (Z-2)	5 × 5min (Z-2)	15min (Z-1)	15min (Z-1)
3 (easy)	2 × 10min (Z-2)	3 × 5min (Z-2)	15min (Z-1)	15min (Z-1)
4 (hard)	3 × 10min (Z-2)	5 × 5min (Z-2)	20min (Z-1)	20min (Z-1)
5 (easy)	2 × 10min (Z-2)	3 × 5min (Z-2)	20min (Z-1)	20min (Z-1)
6 (hard)	3 × 10min (Z-2)	5 × 5min (Z-2)	30min (Z-1)	30min (Z-1)
7 (easy)	2 × 10min (Z-2)	3 × 5min (Z-2)	30min (Z-1)	30min (Z-1)
8 (hard)	2,000m TEST	5 × 5min (Z-2)	2 × 1,000m with 3–5min rest (Z-3)	30min (Z-1)
9 (easy)	10 strokes hard, 20 strokes easy (repeat 6 times)	3 × 5min (Z-2)	30min (Z-1)	30min (Z-1)
10 (hard)	20 strokes hard, 10 strokes easy (repeat 6 times)	5 × 5min (Z-2)	2 × 1,000m with 3–5min rest (Z-3)	30min (Z-1)
11 (easy)	10 strokes hard, 20 strokes easy (repeat 6 times)	3 × 5min (Z-2)	30min (Z-1)	30min (Z-1)

continued opposite

14 Weeks (continued)

Week	Session 1	Session 2	Session 3	Session 4
12 (hard)	20 strokes hard, 10 strokes easy (repeat 6 times)	5 × 5min (Z-2)	2 × 1,000m with 3–5min rest (Z-3)	30min (Z-1)
13 (easy)	10 strokes hard, 20 strokes easy (repeat 6 times)	3 × 5min (Z-2)	20min (Z-1)	20min (Z-1)
14 (race week)	15min (Z-2)	10min (Z-2)	REST	RACE

16 Weeks

Week	Session 1	Session 2	Session 3	Session 4
1 (easy)	2,000m TEST	3 × 5min (Z-2)	10min (Z-1)	10min (Z-1)
2 (hard)	3 × 10min (Z-2)	5 × 5min (Z-2)	15min (Z-1)	15min (Z-1)
3 (easy)	2 × 10min (Z-2)	3 × 5min (Z-2)	15min (Z-1)	15min (Z-1)
4 (hard)	3 × 10min (Z-2)	5 × 5min (Z-2)	20min (Z-1)	20min (Z-1)
5 (easy)	2 × 10min (Z-2)	3 × 5min (Z-2)	20min (Z-1)	20min (Z-1)
6 (hard)	3 × 10min (Z-2)	5 × 5min (Z-2)	30min (Z-1)	30min (Z-1)
7 (easy)	2 × 10min (Z-2)	3 × 5min (Z-2)	30min (Z-1)	30min (Z-1)
8 (hard)	3 × 10min (Z-2)	5 × 5min (Z-2)	2 × 1,000m with 3–5min rest (Z-3)	30min (Z-1)
9 (easy)	2,000m TEST	3 × 5min (Z-2)	30min (Z-1)	30min (Z-1)
10 (hard)	20 strokes hard, 20 strokes easy (repeat 6 times)	5 × 5min (Z-2)	2 × 1,000m with 3–5min rest (Z-3)	30min (Z-1)
11 (easy)	10 strokes hard, 20 strokes easy (repeat 6 times)	3 × 5min (Z-2)	30min (Z-1)	30min (Z-1)
12 (hard)	20 strokes hard, 20 strokes easy (repeat 6 times)	5 × 5min (Z-2)	2 × 1,000m with 3–5min rest (Z-3)	30min (Z-1)
13 (easy)	10 strokes hard, 20 strokes easy (repeat 6 times)	3 × 5min (Z-2)	30min (Z-1)	30min (Z-1)
14 (hard)	20 strokes hard, 20 strokes easy (repeat 6 times)	5 × 5min (Z-2)	3 × 1,000m with 3–5min rest (Z-3)	30min (Z-1)
15 (easy)	10 strokes hard, 20 strokes easy (repeat 6 times)	3 × 5min (Z-2)	20min (Z-1)	20min (Z-1)
16 (race week)	15min (Z-2)	10min (Z-2)	REST	RACE

18 Weeks

Week	Session 1	Session 2	Session 3	Session 4
1 (easy)	2,000m TEST	3 × 5min (Z-2)	10min (Z-1)	10min (Z-1)
2 (hard)	3 × 10min (Z-2)	5 × 5min (Z-2)	15min (Z-1)	15min (Z-1)
3 (easy)	2 × 10min (Z-2)	3 × 5min (Z-2)	15min (Z-1)	15min (Z-1)
4 (hard)	3 × 10min (Z-2)	5 × 5min (Z-2)	20min (Z-1)	20min (Z-1)
5 (easy)	2 × 10min (Z-2)	3 × 5min (Z-2)	20min (Z-1)	20min (Z-1)
6 (hard)	3 × 10min (Z-2)	5 × 5min (Z-2)	30min (Z-1)	30min (Z-1)
7 (easy)	2 × 10min (Z-2)	3 × 5min (Z-2)	30min (Z-1)	30min (Z-1)
8 (hard)	3 × 10min (Z-2)	5 × 5min (Z-2)	2 × 1,000m with 3–5min rest (Z-3)	30min (Z-1)
9 (easy)	2 × 10min (Z-2)	3 × 5min (Z-2)	30min (Z-1)	30min (Z-1)
10 (hard)	2,000m TEST	5 × 5min (Z-2)	2 × 1,000m with 3–5min rest (Z-3)	30min (Z-1)
11 (easy)	10 strokes hard, 20 strokes easy (repeat 6 times)	3 × 5min (Z-2)	30min (Z-1)	30min (Z-1)
12 (hard)	20 strokes hard, 20 strokes easy (repeat 6 times)	5 × 5min (Z-2)	2 × 1,000m with 3–5min rest (Z-3)	30min (Z-1)
13 (easy)	10 strokes hard, 20 strokes easy (repeat 6 times)	3 × 5min (Z-2)	30min (Z-1)	30min (Z-1)
14 (hard)	20 strokes hard, 20 strokes easy (repeat 6 times)	5 × 5min (Z-2)	3 × 1,000m with 3–5min rest (Z-3)	30min (Z-1)
15 (easy)	10 strokes hard, 20 strokes easy (repeat 6 times)	3 × 5min (Z-2)	30min (Z-1)	30min (Z-1)
16 (hard)	20 strokes hard, 20 strokes easy (repeat 6 times)	5 × 5min (Z-2)	3 × 1,000m with 3–5min rest (Z-3)	30min (Z-1)
17 (easy)	10 strokes hard, 20 strokes easy (repeat 6 times)	3 × 5min (Z-2)	20min (Z-1)	20min (Z-1)
18 (race week)	15min (Z-2)	10min (Z-2)	REST	RACE

20 Weeks

Week	Session 1	Session 2	Session 3	Session 4
1 (easy)	2,000m TEST	3 × 5min (Z-2)	10min (Z-1)	10min (Z-1)
2 (hard)	3 × 10min (Z-2)	5 × 5min (Z-2)	15min (Z-1)	15min (Z-1)
3 (easy)	2 × 10min (Z-2)	3 × 5min (Z-2)	15min (Z-1)	15min (Z-1)
4 (hard)	3 × 10min (Z-2)	5 × 5min (Z-2)	20min (Z-1)	20min (Z-1)
5 (easy)	2 × 10min (Z-2)	3 × 5min (Z-2)	20min (Z-1)	20min (Z-1)
6 (hard)	3 × 10min (Z-2)	5 × 5min (Z-2)	30min (Z-1)	30min (Z-1)

continued opposite

20 Weeks (continued)

Week	Session 1	Session 2	Session 3	Session 4
7 (easy)	2 × 10min (Z-2)	3 × 5min (Z-2)	30min (Z-1)	30min (Z-1)
8 (hard)	3 × 10min (Z-2)	5 × 5min (Z-2)	2 × 1,000m with 3–5min rest (Z-3)	30min (Z-1)
9 (easy)	2 × 10min (Z-2)	3 × 5min (Z-2)	30min (Z-1)	30min (Z-1)
10 (hard)	3 × 10min (Z-2)	5 × 5min (Z-2)	2 × 1,000m with 3–5min rest (Z-3)	30min (Z-1)
11 (easy)	2,000m TEST	3 × 5min (Z-2)	30min (Z-1)	30min (Z-1)
12 (hard)	20 strokes hard, 20 strokes easy (repeat 6 times)	5 × 5min (Z-2)	2 × 1,000m with 3–5min rest (Z-3)	30min (Z-1)
13 (easy)	10 strokes hard, 20 strokes easy (repeat 6 times)	3 × 5min (Z-2)	30min (Z-1)	30min (Z-1)
14 (hard)	20 strokes hard, 20 strokes easy (repeat 6 times)	5 × 5min (Z-2)	3 × 1,000m with 3–5min rest (Z-3)	30min (Z-1)
15 (easy)	10 strokes hard, 20 strokes easy (repeat 6 times)	3 × 5min (Z-2)	30min (Z-1)	30min (Z-1)
16 (hard)	20 strokes hard, 20 strokes easy (repeat 6 times)	5 × 5min (Z-2)	3 × 1,000m with 3–5min rest (Z-3)	30min (Z-1)
17 (easy)	10 strokes hard, 20 strokes easy (repeat 6 times)	3 × 5min (Z-2)	30min (Z-1)	30min (Z-1)
18 (hard)	20 strokes hard, 20 strokes easy (repeat 6 times)	5 × 5min (Z-2)	3 × 1,000m with 3–5min rest (Z-3)	30min (Z-1)
19 (easy)	10 strokes hard, 20 strokes easy (repeat 6 times)	3 × 5min (Z-2)	20min (Z-1)	20min (Z-1)
20 (race week)	15min (Z-2)	10min (Z-2)	REST	RACE

22 Weeks

Week	Session 1	Session 2	Session 3	Session 4
1 (easy)	2,000m TEST	3 × 5min (Z-2)	10min (Z-1)	10min (Z-1)
2 (hard)	3 × 10min (Z-2)	5 × 5min (Z-2)	15min (Z-1)	15min (Z-1)
3 (easy)	2 × 10min (Z-2)	3 × 5min (Z-2)	15min (Z-1)	15min (Z-1)
4 (hard)	3 × 10min (Z-2)	5 × 5min (Z-2)	20min (Z-1)	20min (Z-1)
5 (easy)	2 × 10min (Z-2)	3 × 5min (Z-2)	20min (Z-1)	20min (Z-1)
6 (hard)	3 × 10min (Z-2)	5 × 5min (Z-2)	30min (Z-1)	30min (Z-1)
7 (easy)	2 × 10min (Z-2)	3 × 5min (Z-2)	30min (Z-1)	30min (Z-1)
8 (hard)	3 × 10min (Z-2)	5 × 5min (Z-2)	2 × 1,000m with 3–5min rest (Z-3)	30min (Z-1)

continued overleaf

22 Weeks (continued)

Week	Session 1	Session 2	Session 3	Session 4
9 (easy)	2 × 10min (Z-2)	3 × 5min (Z-2)	30min (Z-1)	30min (Z-1)
10 (hard)	3 × 10min (Z-2)	5 × 5min (Z-2)	2 × 1,000m with 3–5min rest (Z-3)	30min (Z-1)
11 (easy)	2 × 10min (Z-2)	3 × 5min (Z-2)	30min (Z-1)	30min (Z-1)
12 (hard)	2,000m TEST	5 × 5min (Z-2)	2 × 1,000m with 3–5min rest (Z-3)	30min (Z-1)
13 (easy)	10 strokes hard, 20 strokes easy (repeat 6 times)	3 × 5min (Z-2)	30min (Z-1)	30min (Z-1)
14 (hard)	20 strokes hard, 20 strokes easy (repeat 6 times)	5 × 5min (Z-2)	3 × 1,000m with 3–5min rest (Z-3)	30min (Z-1)
15 (easy)	10 strokes hard, 20 strokes easy (repeat 6 times)	3 × 5min (Z-2)	30min (Z-1)	30min (Z-1)
16 (hard)	20 strokes hard, 20 strokes easy (repeat 6 times)	5 × 5min (Z-2)	3 × 1,000m with 3–5min rest (Z-3)	30min (Z-1)
17 (easy)	10 strokes hard, 20 strokes easy (repeat 6 times)	3 × 5min (Z-2)	30min (Z-1)	30min (Z-1)
18 (hard)	20 strokes hard, 20 strokes easy (repeat 6 times)	5 × 5min (Z-2)	3 × 1,000m with 3–5min (Z-3)	30min (Z-1)
19 (easy)	10 strokes hard, 20 strokes easy (repeat 6 times)	3 × 5min (Z-2)	30min (Z-1)	30min (Z-1)
20 (hard)	20 strokes hard, 20 strokes easy (repeat 6 times)	5 × 5min (Z-2)	4 × 1,000m with 3–5min rest (Z-3)	30min (Z-1)
21 (easy)	10 strokes hard, 20 strokes easy (repeat 6 times)	3 × 5min (Z-2)	20min (Z-1)	20min (Z-1)
22 (race week)	15min (Z-2)	10min (Z-2)	REST	RACE

24 Weeks

Week	Session 1	Session 2	Session 3	Session 4
1 (easy)	2,000m TEST	3 × 5min (Z-2)	10min (Z-1)	10min (Z-1)
2 (hard)	3 × 10min (Z-2)	5 × 5min (Z-2)	15min (Z-1)	15min (Z-1)
3 (easy)	2 × 10min (Z-2)	3 × 5min (Z-2)	15min (Z-1)	15min (Z-1)
4 (hard)	3 × 10min (Z-2)	5 × 5min (Z-2)	20min (Z-1)	20min (Z-1)
5 (easy)	2 × 10min (Z-2)	3 × 5min (Z-2)	20min (Z-1)	20min (Z-1)
6 (hard)	3 × 10min (Z-2)	5 × 5min (Z-2)	30min (Z-1)	30min (Z-1)
7 (easy)	2 × 10min (Z-2)	3 × 5min (Z-2)	30min (Z-1)	30min (Z-1)

continued opposite

24 Weeks (continued)

Week	Session 1	Session 2	Session 3	Session 4
8 (hard)	3 × 10min (Z-2)	5 × 5min (Z-2)	2 × 1,000m with 3–5min rest (Z-3)	30min (Z-1)
9 (easy)	2 × 10min (Z-2)	3 × 5min (Z-2)	30min (Z-1)	30min (Z-1)
10 (hard)	3 × 10min (Z-2)	5 × 5min (Z-2)	2 × 1,000m with 3–5min rest (Z-3)	30min (Z-1)
11 (easy)	2 × 10min (Z-2)	3 × 5min (Z-2)	30min (Z-1)	30min (Z-1)
12 (hard)	3 × 10min (Z-2)	5 × 5min (Z-2)	2 × 1,000m with 3–5min rest (Z-3)	30min (Z-1)
13 (easy)	2,000m TEST	3 × 5min (Z-2)	30min (Z-1)	30min (Z-1)
14 (hard)	20 strokes hard, 20 strokes easy (repeat 6 times)	5 × 5min (Z-2)	3 × 1,000m with 3–5min (Z-3)	30min (Z-1)
15 (easy)	10 strokes hard, 20 strokes easy (repeat 6 times)	3 × 5min (Z-2)	30min (Z-1)	30min (Z-1)
16 (hard)	20 strokes hard, 20 strokes easy (repeat 6 times)	5 × 5min (Z-2)	3 × 1000m with 3–5min (Z-3)	30min (Z-1)
17 (easy)	10 strokes hard, 20 strokes easy (repeat 6 times)	3 × 5min (Z-2)	30min (Z-1)	30min (Z-1)
18 (hard)	20 strokes hard, 20 strokes easy (repeat 6 times)	5 × 5min (Z-2)	3 × 1000m with 3–5min (Z-3)	30min (Z-1)
19 (easy)	10 strokes hard, 20 strokes easy (repeat 6 times)	3 × 5min (Z-2)	30min (Z-1)	30min (Z-1)
20 (hard)	20 strokes hard, 20 strokes easy (repeat 6 times)	5 × 5min (Z-2)	4 × 1,000m with 3–5min rest (Z-3)	30min (Z-1)
21 (easy)	10 strokes hard, 20 strokes easy (repeat 6 times)	3 × 5min (Z-2)	30min (Z-1)	30min (Z-1)
22 (hard)	20 strokes hard, 20 strokes easy (repeat 6 times)	5 × 5min (Z-2)	4 × 1,000m with 3–5min rest (Z-3)	30min (Z-1)
23 (easy)	10 strokes hard, 20 strokes easy (repeat 6 times)	3 × 5min (Z-2)	20min (Z-1)	20min (Z-1)
24 (race week)	15min (Z-2)	10min (Z-2)	REST	RACE

26 Weeks

Week	Session 1	Session 2	Session 3	Session 4
1 (easy)	2000m TEST	3 × 5min (Z-2)	10min (Z-1)	10min (Z-1)
2 (hard)	3 × 10min (Z-2)	5 × 5min (Z-2)	15min (Z-1)	15min (Z-1)

continued overleaf

26 Weeks (continued)

Week	Session 1	Session 2	Session 3	Session 4
3 (easy)	2 × 10min (Z-2)	3 × 5min (Z-2)	15min (Z-1)	15min (Z-1)
4 (hard)	3 × 10min (Z-2)	5 × 5min (Z-2)	20min (Z-1)	20min (Z-1)
5 (easy)	2 × 10min (Z-2)	3 × 5min (Z-2)	20min (Z-1)	20min (Z-1)
6 (hard)	3 × 10min (Z-2)	5 × 5min (Z-2)	30min (Z-1)	30min (Z-1)
7 (easy)	2 × 10min (Z-2)	3 × 5min (Z-2)	30min (Z-1)	30min (Z-1)
8 (hard)	3 × 10min (Z-2)	5 × 5min (Z-2)	2 × 1,000m with 3–5min rest (Z-3)	30min (Z-1)
9 (easy)	2 × 10min (Z-2)	3 × 5min (Z-2)	30min (Z-1)	30min (Z-1)
10 (hard)	3 × 10min (Z-2)	5 × 5min (Z-2)	2 × 1,000m with 3–5min rest (Z-3)	30min (Z-1)
11 (easy)	2 × 10min (Z-2)	3 × 5min (Z-2)	30min (Z-1)	30min (Z-1)
12 (hard)	3 × 10min (Z-2)	5 × 5min (Z-2)	2 × 1,000m with 3–5min rest (Z-3)	30min (Z-1)
13 (easy)	2 × 10min (Z-2)	3 × 5min (Z-2)	30min (Z-1)	30min (Z-1)
14 (hard)	2000m TEST	5 × 5min (Z-2)	3 × 1,000m with 3–5min rest (Z-3)	30min (Z-1)
15 (easy)	10 strokes hard, 20 strokes easy (repeat 6 times)	3 × 5min (Z-2)	30min (Z-1)	30min (Z-1)
16 (hard)	20 strokes hard, 20 strokes easy (repeat 6 times)	5 × 5min (Z-2)	3 × 1,000m with 3–5min (Z-3)	30min (Z-1)
17 (easy)	10 strokes hard, 20 strokes easy (repeat 6 times)	3 × 5min (Z-2)	30min (Z-1)	30min (Z-1)
18 (hard)	20 strokes hard, 20 strokes easy (repeat 6 times)	5 × 5min (Z-2)	3 × 1,000m with 3–5min (Z-3)	30min (Z-1)
19 (easy)	10 strokes hard, 20 strokes easy (repeat 6 times)	3 × 5min (Z-2)	30min (Z-1)	30min (Z-1)
20 (hard)	20 strokes hard, 20 strokes easy (repeat 6 times)	5 × 5min (Z-2)	4 × 1,000m with 3–5min rest (Z-3)	30min (Z-1)
21 (easy)	10 strokes hard, 20 strokes easy (repeat 6 times)	3 × 5min (Z-2)	30min (Z-1)	30min (Z-1)
22 (hard)	20 strokes hard, 20 strokes easy (repeat 6 times)	5 × 5min (Z-2)	4 × 1,000m with 3–5min rest (Z-3)	30min (Z-1)
23 (easy)	10 strokes hard, 20 strokes easy (repeat 6 times)	3 × 5min (Z-2)	30min (Z-1)	30min (Z-1)
24 (hard)	20 strokes hard, 20 strokes easy (repeat 6 times)	5 × 5min (Z-2)	4 × 1,000m with 3–5min rest (Z-3)	30min (Z-1)
25 (easy)	10 strokes hard, 20 strokes easy (repeat 6 times)	3 × 5min (Z-2)	20min (Z-1)	20min (Z-1)
26 (race week)	15min (Z-2)	10min (Z-2)	REST	RACE

12 Weeks (continued)

Week	Session 1	Session 2	Session 3	Session 4	Session 5
11 (moderate)	20 strokes hard, 15 strokes easy (repeat 7 times)	3 × 7min (Z-2)	3 × 1,500m with 3–5min rest (Z-3)	20min (Z-1)	20min (Z-1)
12 (race week)	20 strokes hard, 15 strokes easy (repeat 6 times)	20min (Z-1)	15min (Z-2)	REST	RACE

14 Weeks

Week	Session 1	Session 2	Session 3	Session 4	Session 5
1 (easy)	2,000m TEST	3 × 6min (Z-2)	3 × 15min (Z-2)	20min (Z-1)	20min (Z-1)
2 (moderate)	3 × 10min (Z-2)	3 × 7min (Z-2)	3 × 15min (Z-2)	20min (Z-1)	20min (Z-1)
3 (hard)	4 × 10min (Z-2)	3 × 8min (Z-2)	3 × 15min (Z-2)	30min (Z-1)	30min (Z-1)
4 (easy)	2 × 10min (Z-2)	3 × 6min (Z-2)	3 × 15min (Z-2)	25min (Z-1)	25min (Z-1)
5 (moderate)	3 × 10min (Z-2)	3 × 7min (Z-2)	3 × 15min (Z-2)	25min (Z-1)	25min (Z-1)
6 (hard)	4 × 10min (Z-2)	3 × 8min (Z-2)	3 × 15min (Z-2)	35min (Z-1)	35min (Z-1)
7 (easy)	2 × 10min (Z-2)	3 × 6min (Z-2)	3 × 15min (Z-2)	30min (Z-1)	30min (Z-1)
8 (moderate)	2,000m TEST	3 × 7min (Z-2)	3 × 1,500m with 3–5min rest (Z-3)	30min (Z-1)	30min (Z-1)
9 (hard)	20 strokes hard, 15 strokes easy (repeat 8 times)	3 × 8min (Z-2)	4 × 1,500m with 3–5min rest (Z-3)	40min (Z-1)	40min (Z-1)
10 (easy)	20 strokes hard, 15 strokes easy (repeat 6 times)	3 × 6min (Z-2)	2 × 1,500m with 3–5min rest (Z-3)	35min (Z-1)	35min (Z-1)
11 (moderate)	20 strokes hard, 15 strokes easy (repeat 7 times)	3 × 7min (Z-2)	3 × 1,500m with 3–5min rest (Z-3)	35min (Z-1)	35min (Z-1)
12 (hard)	20 strokes hard, 15 strokes easy (repeat 8 times)	3 × 8min (Z-2) (Z-3)	4 × 1,500m with 3–5min rest	45min (Z-1)	45min (Z-1)
13 (easy)	20 strokes hard, 15 strokes easy (repeat 6 times)	3 × 6min (Z-2)	2 × 1,500m with 3–5min rest (Z-3)	20min (Z-1)	20min (Z-1)
14 (race week)	20 strokes hard, 15 strokes easy (repeat 6 times)	20min (Z-1)	15min (Z-2)	REST	RACE

16 Weeks

Week	Session 1	Session 2	Session 3	Session 4	Session 5
1 (easy)	2,000m TEST	3 × 6min (Z-2)	3 × 15min (Z-2)	20min (Z-1)	20min (Z-1)
2 (moderate)	3 × 10min (Z-2)	3 × 7min (Z-2)	3 × 15min (Z-2)	20min (Z-1)	20min (Z-1)
3 (hard)	4 × 10min (Z-2)	3 × 8min (Z-2)	3 × 15min (Z-2)	30min (Z-1)	30min (Z-1)
4 (easy)	2 × 10min (Z-2)	3 × 6min (Z-2)	3 × 15min (Z-2)	25min (Z-1)	25min (Z-1)
5 (moderate)	3 × 10min (Z-2)	3 × 7min (Z-2)	3 × 15min (Z-2)	25min (Z-1)	25min (Z-1)
6 (hard)	4 × 10min (Z-2)	3 × 8min (Z-2)	3 × 15min (Z-2)	35min (Z-1)	35min (Z-1)
7 (easy)	2 × 10min (Z-2)	3 × 6min (Z-2)	3 × 15min (Z-2)	30min (Z-1)	30min (Z-1)
8 (moderate)	3 × 10min (Z-2)	3 × 7min (Z-2)	3 × 15min (Z-2)	30min (Z-1)	30min (Z-1)
9 (hard)	2,000m TEST	3 × 8min (Z-2)	4 × 1,500m with 3–5 min rest (Z-3)	40min (Z-1)	40min (Z-1)
10 (easy)	20 strokes hard, 15 strokes easy (repeat 6 times)	3 × 6min (Z-2)	2 × 1,500m with 3–5min rest (Z-3)	35min (Z-1)	35min (Z-1)
11 (moderate)	20 strokes hard, 15 strokes easy (repeat 7 times)	3 × 7min (Z-2)	3 × 1,500m with 3–5min rest (Z-3)	35min (Z-1)	35min (Z-1)
12 (hard)	20 strokes hard, 15 strokes easy (repeat 8 times)	3 × 8min (Z-2)	4 × 1,500m with 3–5min rest (Z-3)	45min (Z-1)	45min (Z-1)
13 (easy)	20 strokes hard, 15 strokes easy (repeat 6 times)	3 × 6min (Z-2)	2 × 1,500m with 3–5min rest (Z-3)	40min (Z-1)	40min (Z-1)
14 (moderate)	20 strokes hard, 15 strokes easy (repeat 7 times)	3 × 7min (Z-2)	3 × 1,500m with 3–5min rest (Z-3)	40min (Z-1)	40min (Z-1)
15 (hard)	20 strokes hard, 15 strokes easy (repeat 8 times)	3 × 8min (Z-2)	4 × 1,500m with 3–5min rest (Z-3)	20min (Z-1)	20min (Z-1)
16 (race week)	20 strokes hard, 15 strokes easy (repeat 6 times)	20min (Z-1)	15min (Z-2)	REST	RACE

18 Weeks

Week	Session 1	Session 2	Session 3	Session 4	Session 5
1 (easy)	2,000m TEST	3 × 6min (Z-2)	3 × 15min (Z-2)	20min (Z-1)	20min (Z-1)
2 (moderate)	3 × 10min (Z-2)	3 × 7min (Z-2)	3 × 15min (Z-2)	20min (Z-1)	20min (Z-1)

continued opposite

18 Weeks (continued)

Week	Session 1	Session 2	Session 3	Session 4	Session 5
3 (hard)	4 × 10min (Z-2)	3 × 8min (Z-2)	3 × 15min (Z-2)	30min (Z-1)	30min (Z-1)
4 (easy)	2 × 10min (Z-2)	3 × 6min (Z-2)	3 × 15min (Z-2)	25min (Z-1)	25min (Z-1)
5 (moderate)	3 × 10min (Z-2)	3 × 7min (Z-2)	3 × 15min (Z-2)	25min (Z-1)	25min (Z-1)
6 (hard)	4 × 10min (Z-2)	3 × 8min (Z-2)	3 × 15min (Z-2)	35min (Z-1)	35min (Z-1)
7 (easy)	2 × 10min (Z-2)	3 × 6min (Z-2)	3 × 15min (Z-2)	30min (Z-1)	30min (Z-1)
8 (moderate)	3 × 10min (Z-2)	3 × 7min (Z-2)	3 × 15min (Z-2)	30min (Z-1)	30min (Z-1)
9 (hard)	4 × 10min (Z-2)	3 × 8min (Z-2)	3 × 15min (Z-2)	40min (Z-1)	40min (Z-1)
10 (easy)	2,000m TEST	3 × 6min (Z-2)	2 × 1,500m with 3–5min rest (Z-3)	35min (Z-1)	35min (Z-1)
11 (moderate)	20 strokes hard, 15 strokes easy (repeat 7 times)	3 × 7min (Z-2)	3 × 1,500m with 3–5min rest (Z-3)	35min (Z-1)	35min (Z-1)
12 (hard)	20 strokes hard, 15 strokes easy (repeat 8 times)	3 × 8min (Z-2)	4 × 1,500m with 3–5min rest (Z-3)	45min (Z-1)	45min (Z-1)
13 (easy)	20 strokes hard, 15 strokes easy (repeat 6 times)	3 × 6min (Z-2)	2 × 1,500m with 3–5min rest (Z-3)	40min (Z-1)	40min (Z-1)
14 (moderate)	20 strokes hard, 15 strokes easy (repeat 7 times)	3 × 7min (Z-2)	3 × 1,500m with 3–5min rest (Z-3)	40min (Z-1)	40min (Z-1)
15 (hard)	20 strokes hard, 15 strokes easy (repeat 8 times)	3 × 8min (Z-2)	4 × 1,500m with 3–5min rest (Z-3)	50min (Z-1)	50min (Z-1)
16 (easy)	20 strokes hard, 15 strokes easy (repeat 6 times)	3 × 6min (Z-2)	2 × 1,500m with 3–5min rest (Z-3)	45min (Z-1)	45min (Z-1)
17 (moderate)	20 strokes hard, 15 strokes easy (repeat 7 times)	3 × 7min (Z-2)	3 × 1,500m with 3–5min rest (Z-3)	20min (Z-1)	20min (Z-1)
18 (race week)	20 strokes hard, 15 strokes easy (repeat 8 times)	20min (Z-1)	15min (Z-2)	REST	RACE

20 Weeks

Week	Session 1	Session 2	Session 3	Session 4	Session 5
1 (easy)	2,000m TEST	3 × 6min (Z-2)	3 × 15min (Z-2)	20min (Z-1)	20min (Z-1)
2 (moderate)	3 × 10min (Z-2)	3 × 7min (Z-2)	3 × 15min (Z-2)	20min (Z-1)	20min (Z-1)

continued overleaf

20 Weeks (continued)

Week	Session 1	Session 2	Session 3	Session 4	Session 5
3 (hard)	4 × 10min (Z-2)	3 × 8min (Z-2)	3 × 15min (Z-2)	30min (Z-1)	30min (Z-1)
4 (easy)	2 × 10min (Z-2)	3 × 6min (Z-2)	3 × 15min (Z-2)	25min (Z-1)	25min (Z-1)
5 (moderate)	3 × 10min (Z-2)	3 × 7min (Z-2)	3 × 15min (Z-2)	25min (Z-1)	25min (Z-1)
6 (hard)	4 × 10min (Z-2)	3 × 8min (Z-2)	3 × 15min (Z-2)	35min (Z-1)	35min (Z-1)
7 (easy)	2 × 10min (Z-2)	3 × 6min (Z-2)	3 × 15min (Z-2)	30min (Z-1)	30min (Z-1)
8 (moderate)	3 × 10min (Z-2)	3 × 7min (Z-2)	3 × 15min (Z-2)	30min (Z-1)	30min (Z-1)
9 (hard)	4 × 10min (Z-2)	3 × 8min (Z-2)	3 × 15min (Z-2)	40min (Z-1)	40min (Z-1)
10 (easy)	2 × 10min (Z-2)	3 × 6min (Z-2)	3 × 15min (Z-2)	35min (Z-1)	35min (Z-1)
11 (moderate)	2,000m TEST	3 × 7min (Z-2)	3 × 1,500m with 3–5min rest (Z-3)	35min (Z-1)	35min (Z-1)
12 (hard)	20 strokes hard, 15 strokes easy (repeat 8 times)	3 × 8min (Z-2)	4 × 1,500m with 3–5min rest (Z-3)	45min (Z-1)	45min (Z-1)
13 (easy)	20 strokes hard, 15 strokes easy (repeat 6 times)	3 × 6min (Z-2)	2 × 1,500m with 3–5min rest (Z-3)	40min (Z-1)	40min (Z-1)
14 (moderate)	20 strokes hard, 15 strokes easy (repeat 7 times)	3 × 7min (Z-2)	3 × 1,500m with 3–5min rest (Z-3)	40min (Z-1)	40min (Z-1)
15 (hard)	20 strokes hard, 15 strokes easy (repeat 8 times)	3 × 8min (Z-2)	4 × 1,500m with 3–5min rest (Z-3)	50min (Z-1)	50min (Z-1)
16 (easy)	20 strokes hard, 15 strokes easy (repeat 6 times)	3 × 6min (Z-2)	2 × 1,500m with 3–5min rest (Z-3)	45min (Z-1)	45min (Z-1)
17 (moderate)	20 strokes hard, 15 strokes easy (repeat 7 times)	3 × 7min (Z-2)	3 × 1,500m with 3–5min rest (Z-3)	45min (Z-1)	45min (Z-1)
18 (hard)	20 strokes hard, 15 strokes easy (repeat 8 times)	3 × 8min (Z-2)	4 × 1,500m with 3–5min rest (Z-3)	55min (Z-1)	55min (Z-1)
19 (easy)	20 strokes hard, 15 strokes easy (repeat 6 times)	3 × 6min (Z-2)	2 × 1,500m with 3–5min rest (Z-3)	20min (Z-1)	20min (Z-1)
20 (race week)	20 strokes hard, 15 strokes easy (repeat 7 times)	20min (Z-1)	15min (Z-2)	REST	RACE

22 Weeks

Week	Session 1	Session 2	Session 3	Session 4	Session 5
1 (easy)	2,000m TEST	3 × 6min (Z-2)	3 × 15min (Z-2)	20min (Z-1)	20min (Z-1)
2 (moderate)	3 × 10min (Z-2)	3 × 7min (Z-2)	3 × 15min (Z-2)	20min (Z-1)	20min (Z-1)
3 (hard)	4 × 10min (Z-2)	3 × 8min (Z-2)	3 × 15min (Z-2)	30min (Z-1)	30min (Z-1)
4 (easy)	2 × 10min (Z-2)	3 × 6min (Z-2)	3 × 15min (Z-2)	25min (Z-1)	25min (Z-1)
5 (moderate)	3 × 10min (Z-2)	3 × 7min (Z-2)	3 × 15min (Z-2)	25min (Z-1)	25min (Z-1)
6 (hard)	4 × 10min (Z-2)	3 × 8min (Z-2)	3 × 15min (Z-2)	35min (Z-1)	35min (Z-1)
7 (easy)	2 × 10min (Z-2)	3 × 6min (Z-2)	3 × 15min (Z-2)	30min (Z-1)	30min (Z-1)
8 (moderate)	3 × 10min (Z-2)	3 × 7min (Z-2)	3 × 15min (Z-2)	30min (Z-1)	30min (Z-1)
9 (hard)	4 × 10min (Z-2)	3 × 8min (Z-2)	3 × 15min (Z-2)	40min (Z-1)	40min (Z-1)
10 (easy)	2 × 10min (Z-2)	3 × 6min (Z-2)	3 × 15min (Z-2)	35min (Z-1)	35min (Z-1)
11 (moderate)	3 × 10min (Z-2)	3 × 7min (Z-2)	3 × 15min (Z-2)	35min (Z-1)	35min (Z-1)
12 (hard)	2,000m TEST	3 × 8min (Z-2)	4 × 1,500m with 3–5min rest (Z-3)	45min (Z-1)	45min (Z-1)
13 (easy)	20 strokes hard, 15 strokes easy (repeat 6 times)	3 × 6min (Z-2)	2 × 1,500m with 3–5min rest (Z-3)	40min (Z-1)	40min (Z-1)
14 (moderate)	20 strokes hard, 15 strokes easy (repeat 7 times)	3 × 7min (Z-2)	3 × 1,500m with 3–5min rest (Z-3)	40min (Z-1)	40min (Z-1)
15 (hard)	20 strokes hard, 15 strokes easy (repeat 8 times)	3 × 8min (Z-2)	4 × 1,500m with 3–5min rest (Z-3)	50min (Z-1)	50min (Z-1)
16 (easy)	20 strokes hard, 15 strokes easy (repeat 6 times)	3 × 6min (Z-2)	2 × 1,500m with 3–5min rest (Z-3)	45min (Z-1)	45min (Z-1)
17 (moderate)	20 strokes hard, 15 strokes easy (repeat 7 times)	3 × 7min (Z-2)	3 × 1,500m with 3–5min rest (Z-3)	45min (Z-1)	45min (Z-1)
18 (hard)	20 strokes hard, 15 strokes easy (repeat 8 times)	3 × 8min (Z-2)	4 × 1,500m with 3–5min rest (Z-3)	55min (Z-1)	55min (Z-1)
19 (easy)	20 strokes hard, 15 strokes easy (repeat 6 times)	3 × 6min (Z-2)	2 × 1,500m with 3–5min rest (Z-3)	50min (Z-1)	50min (Z-1)
20 (moderate)	20 strokes hard, 15 strokes easy (repeat 7 times)	3 × 7min (Z-2)	3 × 1,500m with 3–5min rest (Z-3)	50min (Z-1)	50min (Z-1)

continued overleaf

22 Weeks (continued)

Week	Session 1	Session 2	Session 3	Session 4	Session 5
21 (hard)	20 strokes hard, 15 strokes easy (repeat 8 times)	3 × 8min (Z-2)	4 × 1,500m with 3–5min rest (Z-3)	20min (Z-1)	20min (Z-1)
22 (race week)	20 strokes hard, 15 strokes easy (repeat 6 times)	20min (Z-1)	15min (Z-2)	REST	RACE

24 Weeks

Week	Session 1	Session 2	Session 3	Session 4	Session 5
1 (easy)	2,000m TEST	3 × 6min (Z-2)	3 × 15min (Z-2)	20min (Z-1)	20min (Z-1)
2 (moderate)	3 × 10min (Z-2)	3 × 7min (Z-2)	3 × 15min (Z-2)	20min (Z-1)	20min (Z-1)
3 (hard)	4 × 10min (Z-2)	3 × 8min (Z-2)	3 × 15min (Z-2)	30min (Z-1)	30min (Z-1)
4 (easy)	2 × 10min (Z-2)	3 × 6min (Z-2)	3 × 15min (Z-2)	25min (Z-1)	25min (Z-1)
5 (moderate)	3 × 10min (Z-2)	3 × 7min (Z-2)	3 × 15min (Z-2)	25min (Z-1)	25min (Z-1)
6 (hard)	4 × 10min (Z-2)	3 × 8min (Z-2)	3 × 15min (Z-2)	35min (Z-1)	35min (Z-1)
7 (easy)	2 × 10min (Z-2)	3 × 6min (Z-2)	3 × 15min (Z-2)	30min (Z-1)	30min (Z-1)
8 (moderate)	3 × 10min (Z-2)	3 × 7min (Z-2)	3 × 15min (Z-2)	30min (Z-1)	30min (Z-1)
9 (hard)	4 × 10min (Z-2)	3 × 8min (Z-2)	3 × 15min (Z-2)	40min (Z-1)	40min (Z-1)
10 (easy)	2 × 10min (Z-2)	3 × 6min (Z-2)	3 × 15min (Z-2)	35min (Z-1)	35min (Z-1)
11 (moderate)	3 × 10min (Z-2)	3 × 7min (Z-2)	3 × 15min (Z-2)	35min (Z-1)	35min (Z-1)
12 (hard)	4 × 10min (Z-2)	3 × 8min (Z-2)	3 × 15min (Z-2)	45min (Z-1)	45min (Z-1)
13 (easy)	2,000m TEST	3 × 6min (Z-2)	2 × 1,500m with 3–5min rest (Z-3)	40min (Z-1)	40min (Z-1)
14 (moderate)	20 strokes hard, 15 strokes easy (repeat 7 times)	3 × 7min (Z-2)	3 × 1,500m with 3–5min rest (Z-3)	40min (Z-1)	40min (Z-1)
15 (hard)	20 strokes hard, 15 strokes easy (repeat 8 times)	3 × 8min (Z-2)	4 × 1,500m with 3–5min rest (Z-3)	50min (Z-1)	50min (Z-1)
16 (easy)	20 strokes hard, 15 strokes easy (repeat 6 times)	3 × 6min (Z-2)	2 × 1,500m with 3–5min rest (Z-3)	45min (Z-1)	45min (Z-1)

continued opposite

24 Weeks (continued)

Week	Session 1	Session 2	Session 3	Session 4	Session 5
17 (moderate)	20 strokes hard, 15 strokes easy (repeat 7 times)	3 × 7min (Z-2)	3 × 1,500m with 3–5min rest (Z-3)	45min (Z-1)	45min (Z-1)
18 (hard)	20 strokes hard, 15 strokes easy (repeat 8 times)	3 × 8min (Z-2)	4 × 1,500m with 3–5min rest (Z-3)	55min (Z-1)	55min (Z-1)
19 (easy)	20 strokes hard, 15 strokes easy (repeat 6 times)	3 × 6min (Z-2)	2 × 1,500m with 3–5min rest (Z-3)	50min (Z-1)	50min (Z-1)
20 (moderate)	20 strokes hard, 15 strokes easy (repeat 7 times)	3 × 7min (Z-2)	3 × 1,500m with 3–5min rest (Z-3)	50min (Z-1)	50min (Z-1)
21 (hard)	20 strokes hard, 15 strokes easy (repeat 8 times)	3 × 8min (Z-2)	4 × 1,500m with 3–5min rest (Z-3)	60min (Z-1)	60min (Z-1)
22 (easy)	20 strokes hard, 15 strokes easy (repeat 6 times)	3 × 6min (Z-2)	2 × 1,500m with 3–5min rest (Z-3)	45–60min (Z-1)	45–60min (Z-1)
23 (moderate)	20 strokes hard, 15 strokes easy (repeat 7 times)	3 × 7min (Z-2)	3 × 1,500m with 3–5min rest (Z-3)	20min (Z-1)	20min (Z-1)
24 (race week)	20 strokes hard, 15 strokes easy (repeat 8 times)	20min (Z-1)	15min (Z-2)	REST	RACE

26 Weeks

Week	Session 1	Session 2	Session 3	Session 4	Session 5
1 (easy)	2,000m TEST	3 × 6min (Z-2)	3 × 15min (Z-2)	20min (Z-1)	20min (Z-1)
2 (moderate)	3 × 10min (Z-2)	3 × 7min (Z-2)	3 × 15min (Z-2)	20min (Z-1)	20min (Z-1)
3 (hard)	4 × 10min (Z-2)	3 × 8min (Z-2)	3 × 15min (Z-2)	30min (Z-1)	30min (Z-1)
4 (easy)	2 × 10min (Z-2)	3 × 6min (Z-2)	3 × 15min (Z-2)	25min (Z-1)	25min (Z-1)
5 (moderate)	3 × 10min (Z-2)	3 × 7min (Z-2)	3 × 15min (Z-2)	25min (Z-1)	25min (Z-1)
6 (hard)	4 × 10min (Z-2)	3 × 8min (Z-2)	3 × 15min (Z-2)	35min (Z-1)	35min (Z-1)
7 (easy)	2 × 10min (Z-2)	3 × 6min (Z-2)	3 × 15min (Z-2)	30min (Z-1)	30min (Z-1)
8 (moderate)	3 × 10min (Z-2)	3 × 7min (Z-2)	3 × 15min (Z-2)	30min (Z-1)	30min (Z-1)
9 (hard)	4 × 10min (Z-2)	3 × 8min (Z-2)	3 × 15min (Z-2)	40min (Z-1)	40min (Z-1)

continued overleaf

26 Weeks (continued)

Week	Session 1	Session 2	Session 3	Session 4	Session 5
10 (easy)	2 × 10min (Z-2)	3 × 6min (Z-2)	3 × 15min (Z-2)	35min (Z-1)	35min (Z-1)
11 (moderate)	3 × 10min (Z-2)	3 × 7min (Z-2)	3 × 15min (Z-2)	35min (Z-1)	35min (Z-1)
12 (hard)	4 × 10min (Z-2)	3 × 8min (Z-2)	3 × 15min (Z-2)	45min (Z-1)	45min (Z-1)
13 (easy)	2 × 10min (Z-2)	3 × 6min (Z-2)	3 × 15min (Z-2)	40min (Z-1)	40min (Z-1)
14 (moderate)	2,000m TEST	3 × 7min (Z-2)	3 × 1,500m with 3–5min rest (Z-3)	40min (Z-1)	40min (Z-1)
15 (hard)	20 strokes hard, 15 strokes easy (repeat 8 times)	3 × 8min (Z-2)	4 × 1,500m with 3–5min rest (Z-3)	50min (Z-1)	50min (Z-1)
16 (easy)	20 strokes hard, 15 strokes easy (repeat 6 times)	3 × 6min (Z-2)	2 × 1,500m with 3–5min rest (Z-3)	45min (Z-1)	45min (Z-1)
17 (moderate)	20 strokes hard, 15 strokes easy (repeat 7 times)	3 × 7min (Z-2)	3 × 1,500m with 3–5min rest (Z-3)	45min (Z-1)	45min (Z-1)
18 (hard)	20 strokes hard, 15 strokes easy (repeat 8 times)	3 × 8min (Z-2)	4 × 1,500m with 3–5min rest (Z-3)	55min (Z-1)	55min (Z-1)
19 (easy)	20 strokes hard, 15 strokes easy (repeat 6 times)	3 × 6min (Z-2)	2 × 1,500m with 3–5min rest (Z-3)	50min (Z-1)	50min (Z-1)
20 (moderate)	20 strokes hard, 15 strokes easy (repeat 7 times)	3 × 7min (Z-2)	3 × 1,500m with 3–5min rest (Z-3)	50min (Z-1)	50min (Z-1)
21 (hard)	20 strokes hard, 15 strokes easy (repeat 8 times)	3 × 8min (Z-2)	4 × 1,500m with 3–5min rest (Z-3)	60min (Z-1)	60min (Z-1)
22 (easy)	20 strokes hard, 15 strokes easy (repeat 6 times)	3 × 6min (Z-2)	2 × 1,500m with 3–5min rest (Z-3)	45–60min (Z-1)	45–60min (Z-1)
23 (moderate)	20 strokes hard, 15 strokes easy (repeat 7 times)	3 × 7min (Z-2)	3 × 1,500m with 3–5min rest (Z-3)	45–60min (Z-1)	45–60min (Z-1)
24 (hard)	20 strokes hard, 15 strokes easy (repeat 8 times)	3 × 8min (Z-2)	4 × 1,500m with 3–5min rest (Z-3)	45–60min (Z-1)	45–60min (Z-1)
25 (easy)	20 strokes hard, 15 strokes easy (repeat 6 times)	3 × 6min (Z-2)	2 × 1,500m with 3–5min rest (Z-3)	20min (Z-1)	20min (Z-1)
26 (race week)	20 strokes hard, 15 strokes easy (repeat 7 times)	20min (Z-1)	15min (Z-2)	REST	RACE

Advanced Programmes

Each of the following advanced programmes will alternate between an easy training week and two hard training weeks, to make sure that you get the rest required to perform well and not overtrain. Session six of each week is an optional session, depending on whether or not you have the time that week to train five or six times. If the session involves intervals, you should give yourself from half the interval time up to the full interval time to rest. For example, if a session requires you to row 2 × 4 minutes, then you should give yourself a rest period of 2–4 minutes between each set. Each of the advanced programmes will include two time trials (2,000m test): one at the start of the programme and one halfway through. You should aim for your heart rate to be in Z-3 up to as high as Z-4 (80–100% of your maximum heart rate) for each 2,000m time trial. Time trials are important for gauging how you are improving through the programme, as well as giving you an idea on how to perform on race day. Remember to warm up and cool down with every indoor rowing workout session.

8 Weeks

Week	Session 1	Session 2	Session 3	Session 4	Session 5	Session 6
1 (easy)	2,000m TEST	5 × 5min (Z-2)	3 × 10min (Z-2)	25min (Z-1)	2 × 15min (Z-2)	25min (Z-1)
2 (hard)	30min (Z-1)	5 × 6min (Z-2)	3 × 15min (Z-2)	30min (Z-1)	2 × 20min (Z-2)	30min (Z-1)
3 (hard)	30min (Z-1)	5 × 6min (Z-2)	3 × 15min (Z-2)	30min (Z-1)	2 × 20min (Z-2)	30min (Z-1)
4 (easy)	25min (Z-1)	5 × 5min (Z-2)	3 × 10min (Z-2)	25min (Z-1)	2 × 15min (Z-2)	25min (Z-1)
5 (hard)	2,000m TEST	5 × 6min (Z-2)	1,000m, 750m, 500m, 250m hard with 1min rest between each (repeat 2 times) (Z-3)	3 × 2,000m with 3–5min rest (Z-3)	2 × 20min (Z-2)	35min (Z-1)
6 (hard)	20 strokes hard, 10 strokes easy (repeat 8 times)	5 × 6min (Z-2)	1,000m, 750m, 500m, 250m hard with 1min rest between each (repeat 2 times) (Z-3)	3 × 2,000m with 3–5min rest (Z-3)	2 × 20min (Z-2)	35min (Z-1)
7 (easy)	20 strokes hard, 10 strokes easy (repeat 6 times)	5 × 5min (Z-2)	1,000m, 750m, 500m, 250m hard with 1min rest between each (Z-3)	2 × 2,000m with 3–5min rest (Z-3)	2 × 15min (Z-2)	30min (Z-1)
8 (race week)	20 strokes hard, 10 strokes easy (repeat 6 times)	20min (Z-2)	250m hard with 1min rest (repeat 4 times) (Z-3)	15min (Z-2)	REST	RACE

10 Weeks

Week	Session 1	Session 2	Session 3	Session 4	Session 5	Session 6
1 (easy)	2,000m TEST	5 × 5min (Z-2)	3 × 10min (Z-2)	25min (Z-1)	2 × 15min (Z-2)	25min (Z-1)
2 (hard)	30min (Z-1)	5 × 6min (Z-2)	3 × 15min (Z-2)	30min (Z-1)	2 × 20min (Z-2)	30min (Z-1)
3 (hard)	30min (Z-1)	5 × 6min (Z-2)	3 × 15min (Z-2)	30min (Z-1)	2 × 20min (Z-2)	30min (Z-1)
4 (easy)	25min (Z-1)	5 × 5min (Z-2)	3 × 10min (Z-2)	25min (Z-1)	2 × 15min (Z-2)	25min (Z-1)
5 (hard)	35min (Z-1)	5 × 6min (Z-2)	3 × 15min (Z-2)	35min (Z-1)	2 × 20min (Z-2)	35min (Z-1)
6 (hard)	2,000m TEST	5 × 6min (Z-2)	1,000m, 750m, 500m, 250m hard with 1min rest between each (repeat 2 times) (Z-3)	3 × 2,000m with 3–5min rest (Z-3)	2 × 20min (Z-2)	35min (Z-1)
7 (easy)	20 strokes hard, 10 strokes easy (repeat 6 times)	5 × 5min (Z-2)	1,000m, 750m, 500m, 250m hard with 1min rest between each (Z-3)	2 × 2,000m with 3–5min rest (Z-3)	2 × 15min (Z-2)	30min (Z-1)
8 (hard)	20 strokes hard, 10 strokes easy (repeat 8 times)	5 × 6min (Z-2)	1,000m, 750m, 500m, 250m hard with 1min rest between each (repeat 2 times) (Z-3)	3 × 2,000m with 3–5min rest (Z-3)	2 × 20min (Z-2)	40min (Z-1)
9 (hard)	20 strokes hard, 10 strokes easy (repeat 8 times)	5 × 6min (Z-2)	1,000m, 750m, 500m, 250m hard with 1min rest between each (repeat 2 times) (Z-3)	3 × 2,000m with 3–5min rest (Z-3)	2 × 20min (Z-2)	40min (Z-1)
10 (race week)	20 strokes hard, 10 strokes easy (repeat 6 times)	20min (Z-2)	250m hard with 1min rest (repeat 4 times) (Z-3)	15min (Z-2)	REST	RACE

12 Weeks

Week	Session 1	Session 2	Session 3	Session 4	Session 5	Session 6
1 (easy)	2,000m TEST	5 × 5min (Z-2)	3 × 10min (Z-2)	25min (Z-1)	2 × 15min (Z-2)	25min (Z-1)
2 (hard)	30min (Z-1)	5 × 6min (Z-2)	3 × 15min (Z-2)	30min (Z-1)	2 × 20min (Z-2)	30min (Z-1)
3 (hard)	30min (Z-1)	5 × 6min (Z-2)	3 × 15min (Z-2)	30min (Z-1)	2 × 20min (Z-2)	30min (Z-1)
4 (easy)	25min (Z-1)	5 × 5min (Z-2)	3 × 10min (Z-2)	25min (Z-1)	2 × 15min (Z-2)	25min (Z-1)

continued opposite

12 Weeks (continued)

Week	Session 1	Session 2	Session 3	Session 4	Session 5	Session 6
5 (hard)	35min (Z-1)	5 × 6min (Z-2)	3 × 15min (Z-2)	35min (Z-1)	2 × 20min (Z-2)	35min (Z-1)
6 (hard)	35min (Z-1)	5 × 6min (Z-2)	3 × 15min (Z-2)	35min (Z-1)	2 × 20min (Z-2)	35min (Z-1)
7 (easy)	2,000m TEST	5 × 5min (Z-2)	1,000m, 750m, 500m, 250m hard with 1min rest between each (Z-3)	2 × 2,000m with 3–5min rest (Z-3)	2 × 15min (Z-2)	30min (Z-1)
8 (hard)	20 strokes hard, 10 strokes easy (repeat 8 times)	5 × 6min (Z-2)	1,000m, 750m, 500m, 250m hard with 1min rest between each (repeat 2 times) (Z-3)	3 × 2,000m with 3–5min rest (Z-3)	2 × 20min (Z-2)	40min (Z-1)
9 (hard)	20 strokes hard, 10 strokes easy (repeat 8 times)	5 × 6min (Z-2)	1,000m, 750m, 500m, 250m hard with 1min rest between each (repeat 2 times) (Z-3)	3 × 2,000m with 3–5min rest (Z-3)	2 × 20min (Z-2)	40min (Z-1)
10 (easy)	20 strokes hard, 10 strokes easy (repeat 6 times)	5 × 5min (Z-2)	1,000m, 750m, 500m, 250m hard with 1min rest between each (Z-3)	2 × 2,000m with 3–5min rest (Z-3)	2 × 15min (Z-2)	35min (Z-1)
11 (hard)	20 strokes hard, 10 strokes easy (repeat 8 times)	5 × 6min (Z-2)	1,000m, 750m, 500m, 250m hard with 1min rest between each (repeat 2 times) (Z-3)	3 × 2,000m with 3–5min rest (Z-3)	2 × 20min (Z-2)	30min (Z-1)
12 (race week)	20 strokes hard, 10 strokes easy (repeat 6 times)	20min (Z-2)	250m hard with 1min rest (repeat 4 times) (Z-3)	15min (Z-2)	REST	RACE

14 Weeks

Week	Session 1	Session 2	Session 3	Session 4	Session 5	Session 6
1 (easy)	2,000m TEST	5 × 5min (Z-2)	3 × 10min (Z-2)	25min (Z-1)	2 × 15min (Z-2)	25min (Z-1)
2 (hard)	30min (Z-1)	5 × 6min (Z-2)	3 × 15min (Z-2)	30min (Z-1)	2 × 20min (Z-2)	30min (Z-1)
3 (hard)	30min (Z-1)	5 × 6min (Z-2)	3 × 15min (Z-2)	30min (Z-1)	2 × 20min (Z-2)	30min (Z-1)
4 (easy)	25min (Z-1)	5 × 5min (Z-2)	3 × 10min (Z-2)	25min (Z-1)	2 × 15min (Z-2)	25min (Z-1)
5 (hard)	35min (Z-1)	5 × 6min (Z-2)	3 × 15min (Z-2)	35min (Z-1)	2 × 20min (Z-2)	35min (Z-1)

continued overleaf

14 Weeks (continued)

Week	Session 1	Session 2	Session 3	Session 4	Session 5	Session 6
6 (hard)	35min (Z-1)	5 × 6min (Z-2)	3 × 15min (Z-2)	35min (Z-1)	2 × 20min (Z-2)	35min (Z-1)
7 (easy)	30min (Z-1)	5 × 5min (Z-2)	3 × 10min (Z-2)	30min (Z-1)	2 × 15min (Z-2)	30min (Z-1)
8 (hard)	2,000m TEST	5 × 6min (Z-2)	1,000m, 750m, 500m, 250m hard with 1min rest between each (repeat 2 times) (Z-3)	3 × 2,000m with 3–5min rest (Z-3)	2 × 20min (Z-2)	40min (Z-1)
9 (hard)	20 strokes hard, 10 strokes easy (repeat 8 times)	5 × 6min (Z-2)	1,000m, 750m, 500m, 250m hard with 1min rest between each (repeat 2 times) (Z-3)	3 × 2,000m with 3–5min rest (Z-3)	2 × 20min (Z-2)	40min (Z-1)
10 (easy)	20 strokes hard, 10 strokes easy (repeat 6 times)	5 × 5min (Z-2)	1,000m, 750m, 500m, 250m hard with 1min rest between each (Z-3)	2 × 2,000m with 3–5min rest (Z-3)	2 × 15min (Z-2)	35min (Z-1)
11 (hard)	20 strokes hard, 10 strokes easy (repeat 8 times)	5 × 6min (Z-2)	1,000m, 750m, 500m, 250m hard with 1min rest between each (repeat 2 times) (Z-3)	3 × 2,000m with 3–5min rest (Z-3)	2 × 20min (Z-2)	45min (Z-1)
12 (hard)	20 strokes hard, 10 strokes easy (repeat 8 times)	5 × 6min (Z-2)	1,000m, 750m, 500m, 250m hard with 1min rest between each (repeat 2 times) (Z-3)	3 × 2,000m with 3–5min rest (Z-3)	2 × 20min (Z-2)	45min (Z-1)
13 (easy)	20 strokes hard, 10 strokes easy (repeat 6 times)	5 × 5min (Z-2)	1,000m, 750m, 500m, 250m hard with 1min rest between each (Z-3)	2 × 2,000m with 3–5min rest (Z-3)	2 × 15min (Z-2)	30min (Z-1)
14 (race week)	20 strokes hard, 10 strokes easy (repeat 6 times)	20min (Z-2)	250m hard with 1min rest (repeat 4 times) (Z-3)	15min (Z-2)	REST	RACE

16 Weeks

Week	Session 1	Session 2	Session 3	Session 4	Session 5	Session 6
1 (easy)	2,000m TEST	5 × 5min (Z-2)	3 × 10min (Z-2)	25min (Z-1)	2 × 15min (Z-2)	25min (Z-1)
2 (hard)	30min (Z-1)	5 × 6min (Z-2)	3 × 15min (Z-2)	30min (Z-1)	2 × 20min (Z-2)	30min (Z-1)

continued opposite

16 Weeks (continued)

Week	Session 1	Session 2	Session 3	Session 4	Session 5	Session 6
3 (hard)	30min (Z-1)	5 × 6min (Z-2)	3 × 15min (Z-2)	30min (Z-1)	2 × 20min (Z-2)	30min (Z-1)
4 (easy)	25min (Z-1)	5 × 5min (Z-2)	3 × 10min (Z-2)	25min (Z-1)	2 × 15min (Z-2)	25min (Z-1)
5 (hard)	35min (Z-1)	5 × 6min (Z-2)	3 × 15min (Z-2)	35min (Z-1)	2 × 20min (Z-2)	35min (Z-1)
6 (hard)	35min (Z-1)	5 × 6min (Z-2)	3 × 15min (Z-2)	35min (Z-1)	2 × 20min (Z-2)	35min (Z-1)
7 (easy)	30min (Z-1)	5 × 5min (Z-2)	3 × 10min (Z-2)	30min (Z-1)	2 × 15min (Z-2)	30min (Z-1)
8 (hard)	40min (Z-1)	5 × 6min (Z-2)	3 × 15min (Z-2)	40min (Z-1)	2 × 20min (Z-2)	40min (Z-1)
9 (hard)	2,000m TEST	5 × 6min (Z-2)	1,000m, 750m, 500m, 250m hard with 1min rest between each (repeat 2 times) (Z-3)	3 × 2,000m with 3–5min rest (Z-3)	2 × 20min (Z-2)	40min (Z-1)
10 (easy)	20 strokes hard, 10 strokes easy (repeat 6 times)	5 × 5min (Z-2)	1,000m, 750m, 500m, 250m hard with 1min rest between each (Z-3)	2 × 2,000m with 3–5min rest (Z-3)	2 × 15min (Z-2)	35min (Z-1)
11 (hard)	20 strokes hard, 10 strokes easy (repeat 8 times)	5 × 6min (Z-2)	1,000m, 750m, 500m, 250m hard with 1min rest between each (repeat 2 times) (Z-3)	3 × 2,000m with 3–5min rest (Z-3)	2 × 20min (Z-2)	45min (Z-1)
12 (hard)	20 strokes hard, 10 strokes easy (repeat 8 times)	5 × 6min (Z-2)	1,000m, 750m, 500m, 250m hard with 1min rest between each (repeat 2 times) (Z-3)	3 × 2,000m with 3–5min rest (Z-3)	2 × 20min (Z-2)	45min (Z-1)
13 (easy)	20 strokes hard, 10 strokes easy (repeat 6 times)	5 × 5min (Z-2)	1,000m, 750m, 500m, 250m hard with 1min rest between each (Z-3)	2 × 2,000m with 3–5min rest (Z-3)	2 × 15min (Z-2)	40min (Z-1)
14 (hard)	20 strokes hard, 10 strokes easy (repeat 8 times)	5 × 6min (Z-2)	1,000m, 750m, 500m, 250m hard with 1min rest between each (repeat 2 times) (Z-3)	3 × 2,000m with 3–5min rest (Z-3)	2 × 20min (Z-2)	50min (Z-1)
15 (hard)	20 strokes hard, 10 strokes easy (repeat 8 times)	5 × 6min (Z-2)	1,000m, 750m, 500m, 250m hard with 1min rest between each (repeat 2 times) (Z-3)	3 × 2,000m with 3–5min rest (Z-3)	2 × 20min (Z-2)	30min (Z-1)
16 (race week)	20 strokes hard, 10 strokes easy (repeat 6 times)	20min (Z-2)	250m hard with 1min rest (repeat 4 times) (Z-3)	15min (Z-2)	REST	RACE

18 Weeks

Week	Session 1	Session 2	Session 3	Session 4	Session 5	Session 6
1 (easy)	2,000m TEST	5 × 5min (Z-2)	3 × 10min (Z-2)	25min (Z-1)	2 × 15min (Z-2)	25min (Z-1)
2 (hard)	30min (Z-1)	5 × 6min (Z-2)	3 × 15min (Z-2)	30min (Z-1)	2 × 20min (Z-2)	30min (Z-1)
3 (hard)	30min (Z-1)	5 × 6min (Z-2)	3 × 15min (Z-2)	30min (Z-1)	2 × 20min (Z-2)	30min (Z-1)
4 (easy)	25min (Z-1)	5 × 5min (Z-2)	3 × 10min (Z-2)	25min (Z-1)	2 × 15min (Z-2)	25min (Z-1)
5 (hard)	35min (Z-1)	5 × 6min (Z-2)	3 × 15min (Z-2)	35min (Z-1)	2 × 20min (Z-2)	35min (Z-1)
6 (hard)	35min (Z-1)	5 × 6min (Z-2)	3 × 15min (Z-2)	35min (Z-1)	2 × 20min (Z-2)	35min (Z-1)
7 (easy)	30min (Z-1)	5 × 5min (Z-2)	3 × 10min (Z-2)	30min (Z-1)	2 × 15min (Z-2)	30min (Z-1)
8 (hard)	40min (Z-1)	5 × 6min (Z-2)	3 × 15min (Z-2)	40min (Z-1)	2 × 20min (Z-2)	40min (Z-1)
9 (hard)	40min (Z-1)	5 × 6min (Z-2)	3 × 15min (Z-2)	40min (Z-1)	2 × 20min (Z-2)	40min (Z-1)
10 (easy)	2,000m TEST	5 × 5min (Z-2)	1,000m, 750m, 500m, 250m hard with 1min rest between each (Z-3)	2 × 2,000m with 3–5min rest (Z-3)	2 × 15min (Z-2)	35min (Z-1)
11 (hard)	20 strokes hard, 10 strokes easy (repeat 8 times)	5 × 6min (Z-2)	1,000m, 750m, 500m, 250m hard with 1min rest between each (repeat 2 times) (Z-3)	3 × 2,000m with 3–5min rest (Z-3)	2 × 20min (Z-2)	45min (Z-1)
12 (hard)	20 strokes hard, 10 strokes easy (repeat 8 times)	5 × 6min (Z-2)	1,000m, 750m, 500m, 250m hard with 1min rest between each (repeat 2 times) (Z-3)	3 × 2,000m with 3–5min rest (Z-3)	2 × 20min (Z-2)	45min (Z-1)
13 (easy)	20 strokes hard, 10 strokes easy (repeat 6 times)	5 × 5min (Z-2)	1,000m, 750m, 500m, 250m hard with 1min rest between each (Z-3)	2 × 2,000m with 3–5min rest (Z-3)	2 × 15min (Z-2)	40min (Z-1)
14 (hard)	20 strokes hard, 10 strokes easy (repeat 8 times)	5 × 6min (Z-2)	1,000m, 750m, 500m, 250m hard with 1min rest between each (repeat 2 times) (Z-3)	3 × 2,000m with 3–5min rest (Z-3)	2 × 20min (Z-2)	50min (Z-1)
15 (hard)	20 strokes hard, 10 strokes easy (repeat 8 times)	5 × 6min (Z-2)	1,000m, 750m, 500m, 250m hard with 1min rest between each (repeat 2 times) (Z-3)	3 × 2,000m with 3–5min rest (Z-3)	2 × 20min (Z-2)	50min (Z-1)

continued opposite

18 Weeks (continued)

Week	Session 1	Session 2	Session 3	Session 4	Session 5	Session 6
16 (easy)	20 strokes hard, 10 strokes easy (repeat 6 times)	5 × 5min (Z-2)	1,000m, 750m, 500m, 250m hard with 1min rest between each (Z-3)	2 × 2,000m with 3–5min rest (Z-3)	2 × 15min (Z-2)	45min (Z-1)
17 (hard)	20 strokes hard, 10 strokes easy (repeat 8 times)	5 × 6min (Z-2)	1,000m, 750m, 500m, 250m hard with 1min rest between each (repeat 2 times) (Z-3)	3 × 2,000m with 3–5min rest (Z-3)	2 × 20min (Z-2)	30min (Z-1)
18 (race week)	20 strokes hard, 10 strokes easy (repeat 6 times)	20min (Z-2)	250m hard with 1min rest (repeat 4 times) (Z-3)	15min (Z-2)	REST	RACE

20 Weeks

Week	Session 1	Session 2	Session 3	Session 4	Session 5	Session 6
1 (easy)	2,000m TEST	5 × 5min (Z-2)	3 × 10min (Z-2)	25min (Z-1)	2 × 15min (Z-2)	25min (Z-1)
2 (hard)	30min (Z-1)	5 × 6min (Z-2)	3 × 15min (Z-2)	30min (Z-1)	2 × 20min (Z-2)	30min (Z-1)
3 (hard)	30min (Z-1)	5 × 6min (Z-2)	3 × 15min (Z-2)	30min (Z-1)	2 × 20min (Z-2)	30min (Z-1)
4 (easy)	25min (Z-1)	5 × 5min (Z-2)	3 × 10min (Z-2)	25min (Z-1)	2 × 15min (Z-2)	25min (Z-1)
5 (hard)	35min (Z-1)	5 × 6min (Z-2)	3 × 15min (Z-2)	35min (Z-1)	2 × 20min (Z-2)	35min (Z-1)
6 (hard)	35min (Z-1)	5 × 6min (Z-2)	3 × 15min (Z-2)	35min (Z-1)	2 × 20min (Z-2)	35min (Z-1)
7 (easy)	30min (Z-1)	5 × 5min (Z-2)	3 × 10min (Z-2)	30min (Z-1)	2 × 15min (Z-2)	30min (Z-1)
8 (hard)	40min (Z-1)	5 × 6min (Z-2)	3 × 15min (Z-2)	40min (Z-1)	2 × 20min (Z-2)	40min (Z-1)
9 (hard)	40min (Z-1)	5 × 6min (Z-2)	3 × 15min (Z-2)	40min (Z-1)	2 × 20min (Z-2)	40min (Z-1)
10 (easy)	35min (Z-1)	5 × 5min (Z-2)	3 × 10min (Z-2)	35min (Z-1)	2 × 15min (Z-2)	35min (Z-1)
11 (hard)	2,000m TEST	5 × 6min (Z-2)	1,000m, 750m, 500m, 250m hard with 1min rest between each (repeat 2 times) (Z-3)	3 × 2,000m with 3–5min rest (Z-3)	2 × 20min (Z-2)	45min (Z-1)

continued overleaf

20 Weeks (continued)

Week	Session 1	Session 2	Session 3	Session 4	Session 5	Session 6
12 (hard)	20 strokes hard, 10 strokes easy (repeat 8 times)	5 × 6min (Z-2)	1,000m, 750m, 500m, 250m hard with 1min rest between each (repeat 2 times) (Z-3)	3 × 2,000m with 3–5min rest (Z-3)	2 × 20min (Z-2)	45min (Z-1)
13 (easy)	20 strokes hard, 10 strokes easy (repeat 6 times)	5 × 5min (Z-2)	1,000m, 750m, 500m, 250m hard with 1min rest between each (Z-3)	2 × 2,000m with 3–5min rest (Z-3)	2 × 15min (Z-2)	40min (Z-1)
14 (hard)	20 strokes hard, 10 strokes easy (repeat 8 times)	5 × 6min (Z-2)	1,000m, 750m, 500m, 250m hard with 1min rest between each (repeat 2 times) (Z-3)	3 × 2,000m with 3–5min rest (Z-3)	2 × 20min (Z-2)	50min (Z-1)
15 (hard)	20 strokes hard, 10 strokes easy (repeat 8 times)	5 × 6min (Z-2)	1,000m, 750m, 500m, 250m hard with 1min rest between each (repeat 2 times) (Z-3)	3 × 2,000m with 3–5min rest (Z-3)	2 × 20min (Z-2)	50min (Z-1)
16 (easy)	20 strokes hard, 10 strokes easy (repeat 6 times)	5 × 5min (Z-2)	1,000m, 750m, 500m, 250m hard with 1min rest between each (Z-3)	2 × 2,000m with 3–5min rest (Z-3)	2 × 15min (Z-2)	45min (Z-1)
17 (hard)	20 strokes hard, 10 strokes easy (repeat 8 times)	5 × 6min (Z-2)	1,000m, 750m, 500m, 250m hard with 1min rest between each (repeat 2 times) (Z-3)	3 × 2,000m with 3–5min rest (Z-3)	2 × 20min (Z-2)	55min (Z-1)
18 (hard)	20 strokes hard, 10 strokes easy (repeat 8 times)	5 × 6min (Z-2)	1,000m, 750m, 500m, 250m hard with 1min rest between each (repeat 2 times) (Z-3)	3 × 2,000m with 3–5min rest (Z-3)	2 × 20min (Z-2)	55min (Z-1)
19 (easy)	20 strokes hard, 10 strokes easy (repeat 6 times)	5 × 5min (Z-2)	1,000m, 750m, 500m, 250m hard with 1min rest between each (Z-3)	2 × 2,000m with 3–5min rest (Z-3)	2 × 15min (Z-2)	30min (Z-1)
20 (race week)	20 strokes hard, 10 strokes easy (repeat 6 times)	20min (Z-2)	250m hard with 1min rest (repeat 4 times) (Z-3)	15min (Z-2)	REST	RACE

22 Weeks

Week	Session 1	Session 2	Session 3	Session 4	Session 5	Session 6
1 (easy)	2,000m TEST	5 × 5min (Z-2)	3 × 10min (Z-2)	25min (Z-1)	2 × 15min (Z-2)	25min (Z-1)
2 (hard)	30min (Z-1)	5 × 6min (Z-2)	3 × 15min (Z-2)	30min (Z-1)	2 × 20min (Z-2)	30min (Z-1)
3 (hard)	30min (Z-1)	5 × 6min (Z-2)	3 × 15min (Z-2)	30min (Z-1)	2 × 20min (Z-2)	30min (Z-1)
4 (easy)	25min (Z-1)	5 × 5min (Z-2)	3 × 10min (Z-2)	25min (Z-1)	2 × 15min (Z-2)	25min (Z-1)
5 (hard)	35min (Z-1)	5 × 6min (Z-2)	3 × 15min (Z-2)	35min (Z-1)	2 × 20min (Z-2)	35min (Z-1)
6 (hard)	35min (Z-1)	5 × 6min (Z-2)	3 × 15min (Z-2)	35min (Z-1)	2 × 20min (Z-2)	35min (Z-1)
7 (easy)	30min (Z-1)	5 × 5min (Z-2)	3 × 10min (Z-2)	30min (Z-1)	2 × 15min (Z-2)	30min (Z-1)
8 (hard)	40min (Z-1)	5 × 6min (Z-2)	3 × 15min (Z-2)	40min (Z-1)	2 × 20min (Z-2)	40min (Z-1)
9 (hard)	40min (Z-1)	5 × 6min (Z-2)	3 × 15min (Z-2)	40min (Z-1)	2 × 20min (Z-2)	40min (Z-1)
10 (easy)	35min (Z-1)	5 × 5min (Z-2)	3 × 10min (Z-2)	35min (Z-1)	2 × 15min (Z-2)	35min (Z-1)
11 (hard)	45min (Z-1)	5 × 6min (Z-2)	3 × 15min (Z-2)	45min (Z-1)	2 × 20min (Z-2)	45min (Z-1)
12 (hard)	2,000m TEST	5 × 6min (Z-2)	1,000m, 750m, 500m, 250m hard with 1min rest between each (repeat 2 times) (Z-3)	3 × 2,000m with 3–5min rest (Z-3)	2 × 20min (Z-2)	45min (Z-1)
13 (easy)	20 strokes hard, 10 strokes easy (repeat 6 times)	5 × 5min (Z-2)	1,000m, 750m, 500m, 250m hard with 1min rest between each (Z-3)	2 × 2,000m with 3–5min rest (Z-3)	2 × 15min (Z-2)	40min (Z-1)
14 (hard)	20 strokes hard, 10 strokes easy (repeat 8 times)	5 × 6min (Z-2)	1,000m, 750m, 500m, 250m hard with 1min rest between each (repeat 2 times) (Z-3)	3 × 2,000m with 3–5min rest (Z-3)	2 × 20min (Z-2)	50min (Z-1)
15 (hard)	20 strokes hard, 10 strokes easy (repeat 8 times)	5 × 6min (Z-2)	1,000m, 750m, 500m, 250m hard with 1min rest between each (repeat 2 times) (Z-3)	3 × 2,000m with 3–5min rest (Z-3)	2 × 20min (Z-2)	50min (Z-1)
16 (easy)	20 strokes hard, 10 strokes easy (repeat 6 times)	5 × 5min (Z-2)	1,000m, 750m, 500m, 250m hard with 1min rest between each (Z-3)	2 × 2,000m with 3–5min rest (Z-3)	2 × 15min (Z-2)	45min (Z-1)

continued overleaf

22 Weeks (continued)

Week	Session 1	Session 2	Session 3	Session 4	Session 5	Session 6
17 (hard)	20 strokes hard, 10 strokes easy (repeat 8 times)	5 × 6min (Z-2)	1,000m, 750m, 500m, 250m hard with 1min rest between each (repeat 2 times) (Z-3)	3 × 2,000m with 3–5min rest (Z-3)	2 × 20min (Z-2)	55min (Z-1)
18 (hard)	20 strokes hard, 10 strokes easy (repeat 8 times)	5 × 6min (Z-2)	1,000m, 750m, 500m, 250m hard with 1min rest between each (repeat 2 times) (Z-3)	3 × 2,000m with 3–5min rest (Z-3)	2 × 20min (Z-2)	55min (Z-1)
19 (easy)	20 strokes hard, 10 strokes easy (repeat 6 times)	5 × 5min (Z-2)	1,000m, 750m, 500m, 250m hard with 1min rest between each (Z-3)	2 × 2,000m with 3–5min rest (Z-3)	2 × 15min (Z-2)	50min (Z-1)
20 (hard)	20 strokes hard, 10 strokes easy (repeat 8 times)	5 × 6min (Z-2)	1,000m, 750m, 500m, 250m hard with 1min rest between each (repeat 2 times) (Z-3)	3 × 2,000m with 3–5min rest (Z-3)	2 × 20min (Z-2)	60min (Z-1)
21 (hard)	20 strokes hard, 10 strokes easy (repeat 8 times)	5 × 6min (Z-2)	1,000m, 750m, 500m, 250m hard with 1min rest between each (repeat 2 times) (Z-3)	3 × 2,000m with 3–5min rest (Z-3)	2 × 20min (Z-2)	30min (Z-1)
22 (race week)	20 strokes hard, 10 strokes easy (repeat 6 times)	20min (Z-2)	250m hard with 1min rest (repeat 4 times) (Z-3)	15min (Z-2)	REST	RACE

24 Weeks

Week	Session 1	Session 2	Session 3	Session 4	Session 5	Session 6
1 (easy)	2,000m TEST	5 × 5min (Z-2)	3 × 10min (Z-2)	25min (Z-1)	2 × 15min (Z-2)	25min (Z-1)
2 (hard)	30min (Z-1)	5 × 6min (Z-2)	3 × 15min (Z-2)	30min (Z-1)	2 × 20min (Z-2)	30min (Z-1)
3 (hard)	30min (Z-1)	5 × 6min (Z-2)	3 × 15min (Z-2)	30min (Z-1)	2 × 20min (Z-2)	30min (Z-1)
4 (easy)	25min (Z-1)	5 × 5min (Z-2)	3 × 10min (Z-2)	25min (Z-1)	2 × 15min (Z-2)	25min (Z-1)
5 (hard)	35min (Z-1)	5 × 6min (Z-2)	3 × 15min (Z-2)	35min (Z-1)	2 × 20min (Z-2)	35min (Z-1)
6 (hard)	35min (Z-1)	5 × 6min (Z-2)	3 × 15min (Z-2)	35min (Z-1)	2 × 20min (Z-2)	35min (Z-1)

continued opposite

24 Weeks (continued)

Week	Session 1	Session 2	Session 3	Session 4	Session 5	Session 6
7 (easy)	30min (Z-1)	5 × 5min (Z-2)	3 × 10min (Z-2)	30min (Z-1)	2 × 15min (Z-2)	30min (Z-1)
8 (hard)	40min (Z-1)	5 × 6min (Z-2)	3 × 15min (Z-2)	40min (Z-1)	2 × 20min (Z-2)	40min (Z-1)
9 (hard)	40min (Z-1)	5 × 6min (Z-2)	3 × 15min (Z-2)	40min (Z-1)	2 × 20min (Z-2)	40min (Z-1)
10 (easy)	35min (Z-1)	5 × 5min (Z-2)	3 × 10min (Z-2)	35min (Z-1)	2 × 15min (Z-2)	35min (Z-1)
11 (hard)	45min (Z-1)	5 × 6min (Z-2)	3 × 15min (Z-2)	45min (Z-1)	2 × 20min (Z-2)	45min (Z-1)
12 (hard)	45min (Z-1)	5 × 6min (Z-2)	3 × 15min (Z-2)	45min (Z-1)	2 × 20min (Z-2)	45min (Z-1)
13 (easy)	2,000m TEST	5 × 5min (Z-2)	1,000m, 750m, 500m, 250m hard with 1min rest between each (Z-3)	2 × 2,000m with 3–5min rest (Z-3)	2 × 15min (Z-2)	40min (Z-1)
14 (hard)	20 strokes hard, 10 strokes easy (repeat 8 times)	5 × 6min (Z-2)	1,000m, 750m, 500m, 250m hard with 1min rest between each (repeat 2 times) (Z-3)	3 × 2,000m with 3–5min rest (Z-3)	2 × 20min (Z-2)	50min (Z-1)
15 (hard)	20 strokes hard, 10 strokes easy (repeat 8 times)	5 × 6min (Z-2)	1,000m, 750m, 500m, 250m hard with 1min rest between each (repeat 2 times) (Z-3)	3 × 2,000m with 3–5min rest (Z-3)	2 × 20min (Z-2)	50min (Z-1)
16 (easy)	20 strokes hard, 10 strokes easy (repeat 6 times)	5 × 5min (Z-2)	1,000m, 750m, 500m, 250m hard with 1min rest between each (Z-3)	2 × 2,000m with 3–5min rest (Z-3)	2 × 15min (Z-2)	45min (Z-1)
17 (hard)	20 strokes hard, 10 strokes easy (repeat 8 times)	5 × 6min (Z-2)	1,000m, 750m, 500m, 250m hard with 1min rest between each (repeat 2 times) (Z-3)	3 × 2,000m with 3–5min rest (Z-3)	2 × 20min (Z-2)	55min (Z-1)
18 (hard)	20 strokes hard, 10 strokes easy (repeat 8 times)	5 × 6min (Z-2)	1,000m, 750m, 500m, 250m hard with 1min rest between each (repeat 2 times) (Z-3)	3 × 2,000m with 3–5min rest (Z-3)	2 × 20min (Z-2)	55min (Z-1)
19 (easy)	20 strokes hard, 10 strokes easy (repeat 6 times)	5 × 5min (Z-2)	1,000m, 750m, 500m, 250m hard with 1min rest between each (Z-3)	2 × 2,000m with 3–5min rest (Z-3)	2 × 15min (Z-2)	50min (Z-1)

continued overleaf

24 Weeks (continued)

Week	Session 1	Session 2	Session 3	Session 4	Session 5	Session 6
20 (hard)	20 strokes hard, 10 strokes easy (repeat 8 times)	5 × 6min (Z-2)	1,000m, 750m, 500m, 250m hard with 1min rest between each (repeat 2 times) (Z-3)	3 × 2,000m with 3–5min rest (Z-3)	2 × 20min (Z-2)	60min (Z-1)
21 (hard)	20 strokes hard, 10 strokes easy (repeat 8 times)	5 × 6min (Z-2)	1,000m, 750m, 500m, 250m hard with 1min rest between each (repeat 2 times) (Z-3)	3 × 2,000m with 3–5min rest (Z-3)	2 × 20min (Z-2)	60min (Z-1)
22 (easy)	20 strokes hard, 10 strokes easy (repeat 6 times)	5 × 5min (Z-2)	1,000m, 750m, 500m, 250m hard with 1min rest between each (Z-3)	2 × 2,000m with 3–5min rest (Z-3)	2 × 15min (Z-2)	55min (Z-1)
23 (hard)	20 strokes hard, 10 strokes easy (repeat 8 times)	5 × 6min (Z-2)	1,000m, 750m, 500m, 250m hard with 1min rest between each (repeat 2 times) (Z-3)	3 × 2,000m with 3–5min rest (Z-3)	2 × 20min (Z-2)	30min (Z-1)
24 (race week)	20 strokes hard, 10 strokes easy (repeat 6 times)	20min (Z-2)	250m hard with 1min rest (repeat 4 times) (Z-3)	15min (Z-2)	REST	RACE

26 Weeks

Week	Session 1	Session 2	Session 3	Session 4	Session 5	Session 6
1 (easy)	2,000m TEST	5 × 5min (Z-2)	3 × 10min (Z-2)	25min (Z-1)	2 × 15min (Z-2)	25min (Z-1)
2 (hard)	30min (Z-1)	5 × 6min (Z-2)	3 × 15min (Z-2)	30min (Z-1)	2 × 20min (Z-2)	30min (Z-1)
3 (hard)	30min (Z-1)	5 × 6min (Z-2)	3 × 15min (Z-2)	30min (Z-1)	2 × 20min (Z-2)	30min (Z-1)
4 (easy)	25min (Z-1)	5 × 5min (Z-2)	3 × 10min (Z-2)	25min (Z-1)	2 × 15min (Z-2)	25min (Z-1)
5 (hard)	35min (Z-1)	5 × 6min (Z-2)	3 × 15min (Z-2)	35min (Z-1)	2 × 20min (Z-2)	35min (Z-1)
6 (hard)	35min (Z-1)	5 × 6min (Z-2)	3 × 15min (Z-2)	35min (Z-1)	2 × 20min (Z-2)	35min (Z-1)
7 (easy)	30min (Z-1)	5 × 5min (Z-2)	3 × 10min (Z-2)	30min (Z-1)	2 × 15min (Z-2)	30min (Z-1)
8 (hard)	40min (Z-1)	5 × 6min (Z-2)	3 × 15min (Z-2)	40min (Z-1)	2 × 20min (Z-2)	40min (Z-1)
9 (hard)	40min (Z-1)	5 × 6min (Z-2)	3 × 15min (Z-2)	40min (Z-1)	2 × 20min (Z-2)	40min (Z-1)

continued opposite

26 Weeks (continued)

Week	Session 1	Session 2	Session 3	Session 4	Session 5	Session 6
10 (easy)	35min (Z-1)	5 × 5min (Z-2)	3 × 10min (Z-2)	35min (Z-1)	2 × 15min (Z-2)	35min (Z-1)
11 (hard)	45min (Z-1)	5 × 6min (Z-2)	3 × 15min (Z-2)	45min (Z-1)	2 × 20min (Z-2)	45min (Z-1)
12 (hard)	45min (Z-1)	5 × 6min (Z-2)	3 × 15min (Z-2)	45min (Z-1)	2 × 20min (Z-2)	45min (Z-1)
13 (easy)	40min (Z-1)	5 × 5min (Z-2)	3 × 10min (Z-2)	40min (Z-1)	2 × 15min (Z-2)	40min (Z-1)
14 (hard)	2,000m TEST	5 × 6min (Z-2)	1,000m, 750m, 500m, 250m hard with 1min rest between each (repeat 2 times) (Z-3)	3 × 2,000m with 3–5min rest (Z-3)	2 × 20min (Z-2)	50min (Z-1)
15 (hard)	20 strokes hard, 10 strokes easy (repeat 8 times)	5 × 6min (Z-2)	1,000m, 750m, 500m, 250m hard with 1min rest between each (repeat 2 times) (Z-3)	3 × 2,000m with 3–5min rest (Z-3)	2 × 20min (Z-2)	50min (Z-1)
16 (easy)	20 strokes hard, 10 strokes easy (repeat 6 times)	5 × 5min (Z-2)	1,000m, 750m, 500m, 250m hard with 1min rest between each (Z-3)	2 × 2,000m with 3–5min rest (Z-3)	2 × 15min (Z-2)	45min (Z-1)
17 (hard)	20 strokes hard, 10 strokes easy (repeat 8 times)	5 × 6min (Z-2)	1,000m, 750m, 500m, 250m hard with 1min rest between each (repeat 2 times) (Z-3)	3 × 2,000m with 3–5min rest (Z-3)	2 × 20min (Z-2)	55min (Z-1)
18 (hard)	20 strokes hard, 10 strokes easy (repeat 8 times)	5 × 6min (Z-2)	1,000m, 750m, 500m, 250m hard with 1min rest between each (repeat 2 times) (Z-3)	3 × 2,000m with 3–5min rest (Z-3)	2 × 20min (Z-2)	55min (Z-1)
19 (easy)	20 strokes hard, 10 strokes easy (repeat 6 times)	5 × 5min (Z-2)	1,000m, 750m, 500m, 250m hard with 1min rest between each (Z-3)	2 × 2,000m with 3–5min rest (Z-3)	2 × 15min (Z-2)	50min (Z-1)
20 (hard)	20 strokes hard, 10 strokes easy (repeat 8 times)	5 × 6min (Z-2)	1,000m, 750m, 500m, 250m hard with 1min rest between each (repeat 2 times) (Z-3)	3 × 2,000m with 3–5min rest (Z-3)	2 × 20min (Z-2)	60min (Z-1)
21 (hard)	20 strokes hard, 10 strokes easy (repeat 8 times)	5 × 6min (Z-2)	1,000m, 750m, 500m, 250m hard with 1min rest between each (repeat 2 times) (Z-3)	3 × 2,000m with 3–5min rest (Z-3)	2 × 20min (Z-2)	60min (Z-1)

continued overleaf

26 Weeks (continued)

Week	Session 1	Session 2	Session 3	Session 4	Session 5	Session 6
22 (easy)	20 strokes hard, 10 strokes easy (repeat 6 times)	5 × 5min (Z-2)	1,000m, 750m, 500m, 250m hard with 1min rest between each (Z-3)	2 × 2,000m with 3–5min rest (Z-3)	2 × 15min (Z-2)	55min (Z-1)
23 (hard)	20 strokes hard, 10 strokes easy (repeat 8 times)	5 × 6min (Z-2)	1,000m, 750m, 500m, 250m hard with 1min rest between each (repeat 2 times) (Z-3)	3 × 2,000m with 3–5min rest (Z-3)	2 × 20min (Z-2)	60min (Z-1)
24 (hard)	20 strokes hard, 10 strokes easy (repeat 8 times)	5 × 6min (Z-2)	1,000m, 750m, 500m, 250m hard with 1min rest between each (repeat 2 times) (Z-3)	3 × 2,000m with 3–5min rest (Z-3)	2 × 20min (Z-2)	60min (Z-1)
25 (easy)	20 strokes hard, 10 strokes easy (repeat 6 times)	5 × 5min (Z-2)	1,000m, 750m, 500m, 250m hard with 1min rest between each (Z-3)	2 × 2,000m with 3–5min rest (Z-3)	2 × 15min (Z-2)	30min (Z-1)
26 (race week)	20 strokes hard, 10 strokes easy (repeat 6 times)	20min (Z-2)	250m hard with 1min rest (repeat 4 times) (Z-3)	15min (Z-2)	REST	RACE

Estimated Marathon Pace Based on 5,000m
(Courtesy of Concept2)

5,000m 500m/pace	5,000m time	10,000m 500m/pace	10,000m time	Half marathon 500m/pace	Half marathon time	Marathon 500m/pace	Marathon time
1:30	15:00	1:34	31:20	1:40	1:10:19.4	1:46	2:29:05.3
1:32	15:20	1:36	32:00	1:42	1:11:43.8	1:48	2:31:54.1
1:34	15:40	1:38	32:40	1:45	1:13:50.4	1:51	2:36:07.3
1:36	16:00	1:40	33:20	1:47	1:15:14.8	1:53	2:38:56.1
1:38	16:20	1:42	34:00	1:49	1:16:39.1	1:56	2:43:09.2
1:40	16:40	1:44	34:40	1:51	1:18:03.5	1:58	2:45:58.0
1:42	17:00	1:46	35:20	1:54	1:20:10.1	2:00	2:48:46.8
1:44	17:20	1:49	36:20	1:56	1:21:34.5	2:03	2:53:00.0
1:46	17:40	1:51	37:00	1:58	1:22:58.9	2:05	2:55:48.8

continued opposite

Estimated Marathon Pace Based on 5,000m (continued)

5,000m 500m/pace	5,000m time	10,000m 500m/pace	10,000m time	Half marathon 500m/pace	Half marathon time	Marathon 500m/pace	Marathon time
1:48	18:00	1:53	37:40	2:00	1:24:23.3	2:07	2:58:37.5
1:50	18:20	1:55	38:20	2:02	1:25:47.7	2:10	3:02:50.7
1:52	18:40	1:57	39:00	2:05	1:27:54.2	2:12	3:05:39.5
1:54	19:00	1:59	39:40	2:07	1:29:18.6	2:14	3:08:28:3
1:56	19:20	2:01	40:20	2:09	1:30:43.0	2:17	3:12:41.4
1:58	19:40	2:03	41:00	2:11	1:32:07.4	2:19	3:15:30.2
2:00	20:00	2:05	41:40	2:14	1:34:14.0	2:21	3:18:19.0
2:02	20:20	2:07	42:20	2:16	1:35:38.4	2:24	3:22:32.2
2:04	20:40	2:09	43:00	2:18	1:37:02.8	2:26	3:25:20.9
2:06	21:00	2:11	43:40	2:20	1:38:27.2	2:28	3:28:09.7
2:08	21:20	2:14	44:40	2:22	1:39:51.5	2:31	3:32:22.9
2:10	21:40	2:16	45:20	2:25	1:41:58.1	2:33	3:35:11.7
2:12	22:00	2:18	46:00	2:27	1:43:22.5	2:36	3:39:24.8
2:14	22:20	2:20	46:40	2:29	1:44:46.9	2:38	3:42:13.6
2:16	22:40	2:22	47:20	2:31	1:46:11.3	2:40	3:45:02.4
2:18	23:00	2:24	48:00	2:34	1:48:17.9	2:43	3:49:15.6
2:20	23:20	2:26	48:40	2:36	1:49:42.3	2:45	3:52:04.3
2:22	23:40	2:28	49:20	2:38	1:51:06.7	2:47	3:54:53.1
2:24	24:00	2:30	50:00	2:40	1:52:31.0	2:50	3:59:06.3
2:26	24:20	2:32	50:40	2:42	1:53:55.4	2:52	4:01:55.1
2:28	24:40	2:34	51:20	2:45	1:56:02.0	2:54	4:04:43.9
2:30	25:00	2:36	52:00	2:47	1:57:26.4	2:57	4:08:57.0
2:32	25:20	2:39	53:00	2:49	1:58:50.8	2:59	4:11:45.8
2:34	25:40	2:41	53:40	2:51	2:00:15.2	3:01	4:14:34.6
2:36	26:00	2:43	54:20	2:54	2:02:21:8	3:04	4:18:47.8
2:38	26:20	2:45	55:00	2:56	2:03:46.1	3:06	4:21:36.5
2:40	26:40	2:47	55:40	2:58	2:05:10.5	3:08	4:24:25.3
2:42	27:00	2:49	56:20	3:00	2:06:34.9	3:11	4:28:38.5
2:44	27:20	2:51	57:00	3:02	2:07:59.3	3:13	4:31:27.3
2;46	27:40	2:53	57:40	3:05	2:10:05.9	3:16	4:35:40.4
2:48	28:00	2:55	58:20	3:07	2:11:30.3	3:18	4:38:29.2
2:50	28:20	2:57	59:00	3:09	2:12:54.7	3:20	4:41:18.0
2:52	28:40	2:59	59:40	3:11	2:14:19.1	3:23	4:45:31.2
2:54	29:00	3:01	1:00:20	3:14	2:16:25.6	3:25	4:48:19.9
2:56	29:20	3:04	1:01:20	3:16	2:17:50.0	3:27	4:51:08.7
2:58	29:40	3:06	1:02:00	3:18	2:19:14.4	3:30	4:55:21.9
3:00	30:00	3:08	1:02:40	3:20	2:20:38.8	3:32	4:58:10.7

Marathon Training Programmes

Beginner Programme

The beginner's marathon programme is based over only three indoor rowing sessions each week and alternates between a hard training week and an easy training week. There are no intervals in any workouts throughout this programme because the important goal for beginners is to build up their indoor rowing distance to the point where they can complete the final marathon distance. The final long row of 30,000m should be completed four weeks before the race day, to allow you to reduce the training volume and ensure you are at your fittest on race day. Remember to warm up and cool down, before and after each indoor rowing workout.

Week	Session 1 (Half marathon pace)	Session 2 (Marathon pace)	Session 3 (Marathon pace)
1 (easy)	2,000m	5,000m	7,000m
2 (hard)	3,000m	6,000m	9,000m
3 (easy)	2,000m	4,000m	6,000m
4 (hard)	4,000m	8,000m	12,000m
5 (easy)	3,000m	5,000m	8,000m
6 (hard)	5,000m	10,000m	15,000m
7 (easy)	3,000m	6,000m	9,000m
8 (hard)	6,000m	12,000m	18,000m
9 (easy)	4,000m	7,000m	11,000m
10 (hard)	7,000m	14,000m	21,000m
11 (easy)	4,000m	8,000m	12,000m
12 (hard)	8,000m	16,000m	24,000m
13 (easy)	5,000m	9,000m	14,000m
14 (hard)	9,000m	18,000m	27,000m
15 (easy)	5,000m	10,000m	15,000m
16 (hard)	10,000m	20,000m	30,000m
17 (taper)	9,000m	16,000m	20,000m
18 (taper)	8,000m	12,000m	15,000m
19 (taper)	7,000m	8,000m	10,000m
20 (race week)	5,000m	REST	RACE

Intermediate Programme

The intermediate marathon programme is based on four indoor rowing sessions each week and has an easy training week every third week. Intervals are included throughout the programme to allow you to improve your overall speed over longer distances. The final long row of 32,000m should be completed four weeks before the race day, to allow you to reduce the training volume and ensure you are at your fittest on race day. Remember to warm up and cool down, before and after each indoor rowing workout.

Week	Session 1 (Half marathon pace)	Session 2 (Marathon pace)	Session 3 (Hard week: alternate 5km pace/marathon pace. Easy week: marathon pace)	Session 4 (Marathon pace)
1 (easy)	3,000m	5,000m	4,000m	10,000m
2 (easy)	4,000m	8,000m	4,000m	12,000m
3 (hard)	5,000m	10,000m	1,000m/1,000m (× 2)	14,000m
4 (hard)	6,000m	10,000m	1,000m/1,000m (× 2)	16,000m
5 (easy)	3,000m	6,000m	3,000m	9,000m
6 (hard)	6,000m	12,000m	1,000m/1,000m (× 3)	18,000m
7 (hard)	7,000m	12,000m	1,000m/1,000m (× 3)	20,000m
8 (easy)	4,000m	8,000m	4,000m	11,000m
9 (hard)	7,000m	15,000m	1,500m/1,500m (× 2)	22,000m
10 (hard)	8,000m	15,000m	1,500m/1,500m (× 2)	24,000m
11 (easy)	4,000m	9,000m	4,000m	13,000m
12 (hard)	8,000m	18,000m	1,500m/1,500m (× 3)	26,000m
13 (hard)	9,000m	18,000m	1,500m/1,500m (× 3)	28,000m
14 (easy)	5,000m	10,000m	5,000m	15,000m
15 (hard)	9,000m	20,000m	2,000m/2,000m (× 2)	30,000m
16 (hard)	10,000m	20,000m	2,000m/2,000m (× 2)	32,000m
17 (taper)	9,000m	16,000m	1,000m/1,000m (× 2)	25,000m
18 (taper)	8,000m	12,000m	1,000m/1,000m (× 2)	20,000m
19 (taper)	7,000m	8,000m	1,000m/1,000m (× 2)	15,000m
20 (race week)	5,000m	5,000m	REST	RACE

Advanced Programme

The advanced marathon programme is based on five indoor rowing sessions each week. There is an easy training week every fourth week to allow sufficient recovery and to reduce the risk of injuries. Intervals are included throughout the programme to allow you to improve your overall speed over longer distances. The final long row of 35,000m should be completed four weeks before the race day, to allow you to reduce the training volume, ensuring you are at your fittest on race day. Remember to warm up and cool down, before and after each indoor rowing workout.

Week	Session 1 (Half marathon pace)	Session 2 (Half marathon pace)	Session 3 (Hard week: alternate 5km pace/ marathon pace. Easy week: marathon pace)	Session 4 (Marathon pace)	Session 5 (Marathon pace)
1 (easy)	5,000m	5,000m	8,000m	6,000m	10,000m
2 (hard)	6,000m	6,000m	1,500m/1,500m (× 2)	10,000m	12,000m
3 (hard)	7,000m	7,000m	1,500m/1,500m (× 2)	12,000m	14,000m
4 (hard)	7,000m	7,000m	1,500m/1,500m (× 2)	12,000m	16,000m
5 (easy)	4,000m	4,000m	6,000m	4,000m	9,000m
6 (hard)	7,000m	7,000m	1,500m/1,500m (× 3)	12,000m	18,000m
7 (hard)	8,000m	8,000m	1,500m/1,500m (× 3)	15,000m	20,000m
8 (hard)	8,000m	8,000m	1,500m/1,500m (× 3)	15,000m	22,000m
9 (easy)	5,000m	4,000m	8,000m	5,000m	12,000m
10 (hard)	8,000m	8,000m	2,000m/2,000m (× 2)	15,000m	24,000m
11 (hard)	9,000m	9,000m	2,000m/2,000m (× 2)	18,000m	26,000m
12 (hard)	9,000m	9,000m	2,000m/2,000m (× 2)	18,000m	28,000m
13 (easy)	6,000m	5,000m	9,000m	6,000m	15,000m
14 (hard)	9,000m	9,000m	2,000m/2,000m (× 3)	18,000m	30,000m
15 (hard)	10,000m	10,000m	2,000m/2,000m (× 3)	20,000m	32,000m
16 (hard)	10,000m	10,000m	2,000m/2,000m (× 3)	20,000m	35,000m
17 (taper)	9,000m	9,000m	1,500m/1,500m (× 2)	16,000m	30,000m
18 (taper)	8,000m	8,000m	1,500m/1,500m (× 2)	12,000m	25,000m
19 (taper)	7,000m	7,000m	1,500m/1,500m (× 2)	8,000m	20,000m
20 (race week)	1,000m/1,000m (× 3)	5,000m	5,000m	REST	RACE

Further Reading

Amateur Rowing Association, *Rowing* (Know the Game) (A & C Black Publishers, 2007)

McArthur, J., *High Performance Rowing* (The Crowood Press, 1997)

Nolte, V., *Rowing Faster* (Human Kinetics Publishers, 2005)

Redgrave, S., *Steven Redgrave's Complete Book of Rowing*, 2nd edition (Partridge Press, 1995)

Sandry, C., and J. Shepherd, *Shape Up! Tailor-Made Training for Female Body Shapes* (A & C Black Publishers, 2008)

Shepherd, J., *Shape Up! Tailor-Made Training for Male Body Types* (A & C Black Publishers, 2008)

Index